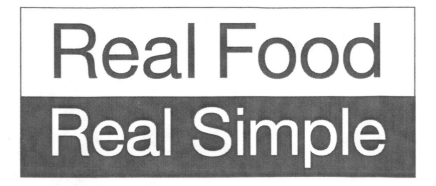

Real Food
Real Simple

A Personalized Plan for More Energy,
Less Stress, and Healthy Meals in Minutes

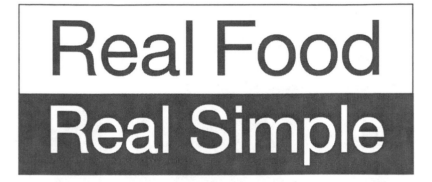

Real Food
Real Simple

A Personalized Plan for More Energy,
Less Stress, and Healthy Meals in Minutes

ERIN HARNER

Real Food, Real Simple
A Personalized Plan for More Energy, Less Stress, and Healthy
Meals in Minutes

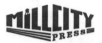

Mill City Press, Inc.
212 3rd Avenue North, Suite 290
Minneapolis, MN 55401
612.455.2294
www.millcitypublishing.com

ISBN-13: 978-1-938008-29-0
LCCN: 2012922951

Cover Design and Typeset by James Arneson

Printed in the United States of America

Author's Note

This book is designed to simplify the vast array of healthy eating information for the reader. It is not intended to review *all* of the information available on the topics of nutrition, health, or food preparation. Much of the research and technical information available was intentionally left out for the sake of simplicity and clarity.

Likewise, this book is not intended to diagnose or treat any condition. If you need medical or other assistance, please seek professional advice. It is recommended that you consult your health-care professional before making changes to your diet. Every effort has been made to make this book as accurate as possible. However, there may be mistakes, both typographical and in content. Therefore, this text should be used as a general guide and not as an ultimate source for health and nutrition information.

Also note that the client stories in this book are all true and only the first names of clients have been used to protect their privacy.

"You don't have to cook fancy or complicated masterpieces—just good food from fresh ingredients." –Julia Child

TABLE OF CONTENTS

The Challenge

"The groundwork of all happiness is health." —James Leigh Hunt

What if you knew exactly what to eat to give you more energy and had a plan to make it work for you every day of the week? How would your life change?

As a society, we're plagued by low energy, endless demands on our time, and health challenge after health challenge. In our country, we've come to accept the fact that this is how it is. We've come to accept mediocrity. We hide behind frumpy clothes and half-hearted attempts at getting healthy and living the life we want, only to fail and return to our old habits.

It's really easy to get sucked into doing what everyone else is doing. After all, "normal" is fat, sick, and tired.

Everywhere you turn, there's a magazine, book, or TV reporter touting the amazing results you'll get when you try the latest fad diet. But with so much contradictory and conflicting information, how do you know what's going to get you through your long, busy days and what's not? When you're already cramming so much into the day, you simply don't have time to sort through all the chaos and confusion, read the scientific literature, and figure out the best food to put in your body.

If you're confused about nutrition and what you should eat, join the club. Nutrition is a fairly young science and as new findings and discoveries are made, recommendations change. For example, in 1912 a Polish biochemist named Casimir Funk discovered vitamins. He thought they were important proteins and coined the term vital amines or "vitamines." Later, researchers realized that vitamins are not proteins and dropped the e. Just one-hundred years ago, we didn't know what vitamins were or their function in the body.

The fields of nutrition and health are rapidly changing, but one thing that hasn't changed in the past several centuries is food—real food. (Well, it has and it hasn't but we'll get to that.) Real food is whole and natural. It is a product of nature, not industry. Real food is not processed and is easy to recognize because it doesn't come out of a box, bag, can, or other type of package. Vegetables, fruits, whole grains, beans and legumes, nuts and seeds, meat, poultry, seafood, dairy, eggs, herbs, and spices are all real food.

In response to the latest nutritional breakthrough or our innate desire to try something new, fad diets have become unbelievably popular. When they don't work, there are a lot more to try, so we keep dieting. Fad diets place a strong emphasis on counting calories, counting carbs, fat grams, grams of protein, good carbs versus bad carbs, and so on. They focus more on what you *can't* have than what you can. They may work in the short term, but most diets aren't long-term solutions. Diets are something you go on for a period of time, but as soon as you veer from the often superstrict eating plan, you bounce back to your previous weight or sometimes even become heavier than you were previously.

The fad diet of the day just isn't going to cut it. There is a big difference between "going on a diet" and having a diet. Eating a diet made up of real food is not dieting. This is not some short-term quick fix. Eating real food involves adding healthy foods into your diet and crowding out the health-depleting junk. It does not involve deprivation, starvation, or a feeling of missing out like most "diets" do. Consuming a health-promoting real-food diet is a long-lasting and lifelong process. For the rest of this book, consider the word "diet" to simply mean what you eat.

If you really want more energy, to reach and maintain your optimal weight, to feel great in your body, and to achieve more in life than just making it through the day without crashing, then it is time to take a serious look at what you are putting in your mouth. Nothing will make you sick or make you well like food will—specifically, eating real food.

If you aren't happy with your current health level, it's not your fault. There are several huge things working against you, and unless you can see them for what they are and knowingly choose another path, your health will not change.

The first enormous challenge is time and ever-increasing demands on your schedule. If you don't make health a priority, you won't find time for it. The day-in and day-out routine of your busy life takes its toll on your physical well-being. Being constantly on the go with little downtime puts a lot of stress on the body. Believe it or not, when your body senses stress, it literally sends out chemicals to store fat and crave sugar. Your body is told that life is an emergency, and it prepares for the worst. This is an evolutionary survival mechanism and a critical warning sign that many people ignore. When you ignore your body and eat sugar or caffeine to give you a boost when you're exhausted, you take a ride on the blood-sugar roller coaster. When you go up and down and up and down, the end result is exhaustion.

There are two other circumstances where you may be putting chronic stress on your body without giving it much thought. Eating a poor diet full of processed foods puts added stress on the body because it has to digest and absorb the food you're eating. Processed foods filled with sugar and salt take a toll on the body organs, creating stress from the inside as these organs attempt to assimilate these unnatural foods. Another form of stress is caused when you're not getting *enough* nutrition. The body needs the macronutrients (carbohydrates, protein, and fat) as well as the micronutrients (vitamins, and minerals) to function properly. If you're missing a nutrient that the body needs, it has to make up for it somehow and is forced to work harder and less efficiently. So in essence, eating junk food creates a stress response in your body whether you are aware of it or not.

Beyond the stress response created by a poor diet or lack of nutrition, another thing you're up against is your evolutionary inclination to eat fat and sugar. In the hunter-gatherer era, craving fat and sugar kept us alive. But there were no supermarkets, fast-food chains, or manufacturing plants back then. The overall availability of food and the types of food we eat has changed so much in such a short time that our bodies are having a really hard time keeping up with the pace of processed-food manufacturers. If you were to plot the longevity of the highly processed food that humans eat today on a one-year scale of human history, our modern diet would be about two seconds. We are not eating what our bodies were meant to eat, and our health and energy are suffering as a result. Just think of the diet of most Americans: a carb-loaded breakfast, junk food for lunch, and whatever is prepared or easy for dinner. The modern convenience-driven diet is composed mostly of processed food-like substances, and it is a big problem.

But this lifestyle is hard to avoid. The multibillion-dollar processed-food industry consistently blasts you with commercials, ads, packaging, health claims, and other marketing messages to get you to buy and consume their products. They keep doing it because it works. Processed food and fast food is cheap and convenient, and unfortunately, the producers of this food have the money to project hundreds of messages at us every day telling us that that is what we should be eating.

When you combine the increasing demands on your time with convenient meals and snacks, it's easy to get tricked into thinking that eating out three meals per day and grabbing quick snacks from the vending machine, bakery, or coffee shop is actually a good idea.

But with so little free time throughout the day, what are the options? This leads to the bigger challenge, which is that, as a society, we simply don't know how to put quick, simple, healthy, and delicious meals on the table. Cooking healthy meals from scratch went out the window with the processed-food revolution after World War II. We never learned how to cook or prepare meals at home and are often forced to rely on processed food and fast food instead. And let's be honest, those healthy meals of the past sometimes took all day to prepare. Nowadays, if you don't have a strategy that works to make preparing and eating healthy meals simple and quick, it's not going to happen. The main purpose of this book is to give you a strategy that works every time.

Despite all of these challenges, you likely know what healthy food is and probably have a good idea about what eating healthy means. The challenge is actually doing it. The fact is, you have two choices. You can blame yourself for your lack of willpower, while ignoring the enormous external triggers and the fact that the habits you've established are sabotaging your best intentions and well-laid plans. Or, you can bring your habits to the surface by becoming aware of what you're doing and eating and focus your time and energy on creating new habits and practices that work for you.

Despite your best intentions, when life gets busy, you resort to what you know. W. L. Bateman said, "If you keep on doing what you've always done, you'll keep on getting what you've always got." In order to be healthy, you need to change what you do and what you eat each day. The things you do each day automatically comprise your "daily routine" or your habits. What you're going to learn in this book is how to upgrade your choices and modify your habits so you become healthy and do healthy things out of habit. According to the Encarta English Dictionary, the word *habit* means, "an action or pattern of behavior that is repeated so often that it becomes typical of somebody, although he or she may be unaware of it."

So if you've noticed that your eating habits have slipped, it's time to think about changing those habits and eating differently.

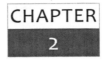

Change Your Eating Habits, Change Your Life

"Those who think they have no time for healthy eating will sooner or later have to find time for illness." –Edward Stanley

After working with clients for several years in my private nutrition-coaching practice to help them improve their diets and conquer health challenges, I had a major realization. It wasn't that my clients didn't know what healthy eating meant or what foods were better than others. They had a general idea, and you do too. What I realized is that there is a giant gap and often a giant leap of faith that you must take to transition from eating the same processed-food diet that everyone else is eating to putting healthy real-food meals on the table.

In this book, I'm going to ask you to step up to radically change your life and improve your health. You may feel like setting up your kitchen, meal planning, shopping for healthy foods, and preparing meals at home is a lot more work than what you are currently doing or what others are doing, but hear me out, because the rewards are incredible. Remember that "normal" is fat, sick, and tired. If you truly want more energy, less stress, and healthy meals in minutes, you're going to have to go against the grain of what most people are doing.

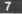

Food is fuel, and every single bite or sip that you eat, digest, and absorb becomes your skin, muscles, fat, hair, brain ... everything. Your food becomes *you!* As a result, eating real food nourishes your body. Feeding your family healthy meals nourishes them. When your bodies are nourished, you have a lot more energy, vitality, and a healthy glow. You have more self-confidence and you feel good. This allows you to get more done and enjoy life to a greater degree.

The whole point of eating is to create energy. Food is made up of nutrients and calories. Each calorie is literally a unit of energy. The definition of *energy* is "the ability to do work." Physical work or mental work, it doesn't matter—when you eat, you should gain energy from the food you eat, period. If the food you eat does not give you energy, you've got a big problem.

When you eat real food, it converts to clean energy in your body. Junk food undergoes the same type of conversion, but the result is very different. One nourishes and the other depletes the body. To think about this another way, if you put the right kind of gas in your car, it should run. If you put fuel in your body, it should run and not get tired, achy, crampy, or anything else. Fueling up at McDonald's is like putting diesel in a gas engine—the fuel is too dirty for the engine to run properly, and it will malfunction. Don't let this happen to you.

When you eat a diet full of nutrient-dense foods, all the other things you're supposed to watch out for—calories, grams of fat, grams of carbs, cholesterol, sodium—become entirely irrelevant. It's time to ditch the diet mentality and embrace a more healthful pattern of eating.

But before you can make that transition and begin to improve, you have to know exactly where you are and acknowledge it.

Wherever you are, it's all good. If you're ten pounds overweight, own it. If you're thirty pounds overweight, acknowledge that it's where you are. If your acne keeps coming back despite trying all the creams and potions, know that you're in the right place. When you're bored, tired, or frustrated and the first place you go is the fridge, it's okay. If your kids drink soda and eat candy more than once a week, that's the situation. Just know that in all the aforementioned situations, there is room for improvement.

Take a moment to acknowledge where you are. What are some of your health challenges? What do you want to improve? What do you want to change or do differently? When you make some changes and embrace being healthy, how will that make you feel?

Just because you are where you are, doesn't mean you have to stay there any longer. The decisions you've made in the past led to you being here today. Wherever you are, be kind to yourself. Don't rip yourself apart for making some poor decisions along the way.

Humans are creatures of habit. We tend to do the same thing each day whether we acknowledge that we do it or not. Your daily routine or collection of habits throughout the day can either work to your demise or you can incorporate healthy habits to make it work to your advantage. The key is to make a plan to create a healthy food environment, where eating healthy real-food meals is the simple, easy, and obvious choice for you.

Aristotle once said, "We are what we repeatedly do. Excellence, then, is not an act, but a habit." If you want excellent health and to feel awesome in your body, you need to repeatedly do good things for yourself. This includes shopping for fresh food and preparing, cooking, and eating healthy and nourishing meals every day. The advantage you have going for you is that you already eat three to six times per day. Because of this, all you need to do is upgrade some of the things you're already doing so you can piggy-back new habits on ones you've already created. This makes incorporating new habits into your life much easier.

One problem is that we rarely stop to evaluate the things we do on a daily basis and ask, "Is this thing I do every day serving me?" There are some things that you do every single day that don't make any sense. And I'm sure there are also habits that you've incorporated into your life every day that serve you well.

If health is truly one of your priorities, reassessing your habits is critical. Grab a piece of paper, and as you continue throughout your day, write down things that you do automatically without even thinking about them. It could include showering, brushing your teeth, skipping breakfast, stopping at Starbucks for your morning latte, eating an apple midmorning, a hamburger and fries for lunch in the cafeteria at work, taking the stairs, and so on.

Don't judge what you do, just write it down. Remember, you have to acknowledge where you are currently before you can begin to improve upon it. You've adopted this daily routine, and the easiest way to improve it to serve your goals and reflect your priorities is to know what you do automatically, without thinking about it. These automatic actions are one reason that most diets fail—we sabotage our efforts without even knowing it!

Doing this requires an open mind and a willingness to change. Change is hard. Doing things differently takes effort at first, and then those new things become habit. Also, when it comes to changing your diet, there is often an element of fear of the un-known. What does kale taste like it? Will I like it? How do you make it? Can you put it in soup? The faster you can tackle these fears and just start trying new foods, the faster you will radically improve your health, boost your energy, gain a renewed sense of confidence in the kitchen, and begin forming healthy habits. What do you have to lose? Excess weight? Belly fat? A health-deteriorating diet? Bad habits?

This book is all about implementing practical strategies that fit your schedule and your lifestyle. You're going to learn the why, the what, and the how of making real food fit into your life, no matter your situation. Strategies don't work unless they are immediately useful and make it easy to incorporate what you're already doing. We're going to do both.

Get Fired Up and Take Action

"Action expresses priorities." –Mahatma Gandhi

Only when you have a strong desire to do something, will you actually do it. A strong reason will drive a strong motivation to take action, and you will be inspired to make some major changes to your habits and diet. This chapter will get you fired up with a mind-set for success. Also, if you're hesitant or not sure about making changes or taking on something new, we're going to put your mind to rest.

If you're thinking that you're already busy or cannot find time to make real lasting changes to your diet, you are not alone. The truth is that it's not a matter of how busy you are, it's much more a matter of how you choose to spend your time.

Whatever is important to you is what you should focus on. Priorities equal focus. Without priorities, we end up scattered, frustrated, and rarely get where we want to go. Let's make this very clear—if your health is not on your list of priorities, you will not get healthy. What you focus on in a positive way expands, and what you ignore contracts. So if you want your health to grow, quite simply you need to make it a priority and focus on improving it, then consistently take positive action.

When is the last time you wished for more time? I hear it every day: "If only I had another couple hours to do this." We all get twenty-four hours in a day. Healthy people plan how they will spend their time and proceed to follow the plan carefully. Unhealthy people fritter away their time at work, in front of the TV, or doing mindless activities like reading status updates on Facebook.

Since we all get the same gift of time, if you want to do more in the time you have the best possible thing to do is raise your energy level. More energy comes from improving your health, nourishing your body and your mind, and paying close attention to your food and nutrition (where your energy actually comes from). If you had more energy, you could get a lot more done in less time, right? This book will show you how to do just that—raise your energy by making a plan to nourish your body with real food.

Doing something different and making a change can be really scary, though. We put up a lot of resistance to change both consciously and subconsciously. Resistance is often a result of fear. "What will my family think if I start serving salmon or quinoa at dinner?" All these "what ifs" keep you stuck. When you acknowledge your fear, quit analyzing what everyone else will think, and decide to change—magic happens. When you step outside of your comfort zone and change your eating habits, you will start feeling how you want to feel—energetic, enthusiastic, radiant, and alive.

But altering your lifestyle can be conceptually scary in and of itself. How should you start? Creating change is a lot easier and faster if you focus on the things that make the biggest impact. Also known as the 80-20 Rule, Pareto's Principle holds some serious power if you understand how it impacts your life. Basically, the 80-20 Rule states that you get 80 percent of the results from only 20 percent of the effort. Conversely, you only get 20 percent of the results from 80 percent of the things you do.

You may have heard about Pareto's Principle as it applies to your closet—you wear 20 percent of your clothes 80 percent of the time. If you don't believe it, go take a look through your closet and sort your clothes into the well-worn 20 percent and little-worn 80 percent.

Here are some ultra-powerful applications of the 80-20 rule to food and nutrition. You eat the same 20 foods 80 percent of the time. What if you upgraded some of those 20 foods to healthy real-food alternatives? You could swap romaine lettuce for iceberg lettuce, whole-wheat pasta or spaghetti squash for white pasta, brown rice for white rice, or an apple for apple juice.

Also, you make the same 20 meals 80 percent of the time. What if you upgraded the ingredients or how you prepare some of those 20 meals that you eat over and over again? By making simple real-food upgrades to what you're already eating on a regular basis, upgrading your diet to a real-food diet becomes a whole lot easier.

You learned from the 80-20 Rule that 20 percent of your choices or effort creates 80 percent of your results. By focusing on the 20 percent that really makes a difference and letting go of your need to get everything perfect or "just right," you will make progress much more quickly. Good enough is really good enough.

On the flip side, focusing on perfection often forces you to procrastinate and creates a lot of stress. You overthink and analyze and overanalyze everything. When you focus on having a "perfect diet" or "perfect dinner" or "perfect abs" or "perfect anything," you stop yourself before you even start, because you know it will never be perfect. Instead of embracing imperfection and "good enough," you never even get started. Perfection does not serve you. Let it go.

So go ahead, burn the rice. Watch your quinoa turn to mush when you stir it instead of just letting it be. Mismeasure the amount of water in your buckwheat pancakes. It's okay! When you try something new, most of the time you won't be good at it the first time you do it. Every time you try something new, you will learn what to do and what not to do. It's not the end of the world if you make a mistake. I've actually created some pretty fabulous new recipes because I screwed something up.

Keep in mind that this book is all about eating real food. What it's not about is processed-food perfection or turning into a real-food dictator. Trying to be perfect with your diet and avoiding all food-like substances (non–real foods) is just not reality. There is no such thing as the perfect diet. It doesn't exist. Your quest for it will drive you and everyone around you nuts. Instead, aim for 90 percent real food and 10 percent other stuff. 95 and 5 percent works great, too. Eat clean most of the time, and the other small percent of the time, live it up. Have a small piece of your daughter's birthday cake or have a glass of red wine with dinner.

Use whatever ratio feels good to you as long as it's not 100 percent and 0 percent. When it comes to meals and snacks, eating clean 100 percent of the time is a surefire recipe for disaster and why you probably tried some diets in the past that you couldn't stick to for more than a few days. When you have absolutely no wiggle room and you have a treat (and you will have a treat), you blow your "diet." You fall off the wagon. And this spirals into a whirlwind of self-criticism and self-loathing. You convince yourself that you can't stick to anything. You say and feel horrible things about yourself. You tear yourself to bits and are so hard on yourself that you quit feeling like you will ever succeed, so you stop trying.

Quit striving for perfection, and you will set yourself up to succeed. Cultivate a beginner's mind, instead. The beginner is eager to learn and open to new ideas and new ways of doing things. Cut yourself some slack as you incorporate new healthy habits into your life. It won't ever be perfect, but keep practicing, and you will get better and faster each time.

Having a clear outcome in mind and taking the steps to make that outcome your reality is really powerful. If you don't determine the results you want first, it's hard to make a plan. So what do you want to achieve? Yes, that is a question. Go ahead—take a few minutes to write down your answer. Do these things that you want to achieve have a timeframe and a clear outcome? Without a goal to strive for, you are directionless and will find it difficult to stay on track and finish what you start.

Don't worry about how you're going to make your health and nutrition goals happen yet. That is where the plan comes in and what the rest of the book is about. I'm going to show you how to make healthy eating a reality in the pages of this book, whether you're at home or not.

Make a decision to achieve your goals. Decide to succeed no matter what. Life comes up. Things come up. We get busy and forget what's important, what we're striving for, and why. We lose sight of the outcome and how we'll feel when we succeed. Too often, you give up when you're 98 percent of the way to achieving your goal. Don't let this happen to you. Follow through. When you set goals and follow through until they are complete, you'll learn to start trusting yourself again.

One big key to finishing what you start is to take small steps. Don't try to tackle everything at once like cleaning out your kitchen and pantry, buying new ingredients, making new recipes for every meal, and replacing your cookbooks with healthier options all at the same time. This all-or-nothing approach works for some but is likely to overwhelm you to the point of quitting. Don't let this happen. Take small steps and make progress one project or new thing at a time, or enlist a coach, a friend, or a family member to help keep you motivated. This is why I coach clients over a period of time from two months to six months, so they have time to integrate what they learn into their diets and into their lives. Having a mentor, support, and accountability really helps them stay on track.

I've read too many self-help books, however, to not be skeptical about the viability of achieving an outcome, and this book is no exception. You can read this book, get some great ideas, and ... well ... just fill your head with great ideas. Do not let this happen. This is a get-up-and-get-going book. I'm going to ask you to step up and actually *do it*. Sometimes you just have to quit learning and start doing. I'm a huge fan of just-in-time learning. If you're reading this, you're just in time.

Success in anything comes to those who take consistent action. Instead of just reading this book, actually do the actions in each section in order. That way, instead of just *learning* how to plan for, shop for, prepare, and eat healthy food, when you finish this book, you will actually be *doing* it. Consuming a diet filled with fresh real food takes planning, practice, and persistence. Eating real food has a learning curve, but the benefits far outweigh the time and effort required to make it happen.

One word of caution—we live in a left-brain society. It's the adult thing to do to make logical, well-thought-out decisions, right? Yeah—sometimes. That assumption has gotten me into trouble more times than I can count on my fingers and toes. We've disconnected our heads from our hearts and our bodies. Making choices with your head is great in certain situations. Which type of jam should I buy? The all-fruit, the organic sweetened with fruit juice, or the store brand loaded with sugar? Does the increased cost justify the benefits of reducing my sugar intake? We ask ourselves questions like these all the time. Given what we know, what we want, and our budget, we make logical decisions.

Here's the thing—our gut is our second brain, and we need to listen to it more often. You have the mysterious "sixth sense" called *intuition*. According to the Encarta English Dictionary, intuition is "instinctive knowledge" or "the state of being aware of or knowing something without having to discover or perceive it." That's pretty cool. When you tap into your intuition and reconnect what you feel with what you think and how you make decisions, you will experience true nourishment. As you dig into making changes to your diet and create a personalized real-food nutrition plan, be very conscious of what "feels right" and what "feels off." If you try a new food that makes you feel awesome and replace that food in your diet for something you were eating before that zaps your energy, you will create a shift. The only way you would know whether a food makes you feel awesome or drains your energy, however, is to trust your body, go with your gut, and pay attention.

Most of the time, you won't know if something is going to work or not until you try it out. So try it. Give it a go, and see if it works for you. If you try it in a few different recipes and decide that you just don't like millet, at least you tried it, and now you know not to buy it or make it again.

When you get inspired to do something, do it. Excitement is temporary. I'm not talking about running around following your folly from one thing to another or chasing bright, shiny objects. If that's all you did, you'd probably have a lot a fun but not really get where you want to go. Many of us follow our impulses, which is not all that different from following our folly. You have an impulse to buy something, so you buy it. You use it for a bit and then forget about it. When the next bright shiny object (or fad diet) appears, you move on to that until you get sick of it and move on. We act like two-year-olds playing with their toys.

When the initial rush of enthusiasm strikes, life is good. You run like the wind. Then life happens, and you stop running. You either quit entirely or you slow down enough to lose interest. Instead, follow your plan and keep making small steps toward achieving your goals. By doing this, you will experience quick wins. It will pump you up, and you'll want to continue making changes. This momentum will keep you moving forward and taking consistent action.

CHAPTER
4

What Real Food Is

"Eat food. Not too much. Mostly plants." –Michael Pollan

Understanding what real food is is the key to building a healthy foundation of true health and outrageous energy. What you're going to learn in this book about real food can be applied to your diet (what you eat), whatever you choose it to be. Whether you eat gluten-free, dairy-free, vegetarian, vegan, seafood but no meat, raw foods, grain-free, or whatever, it doesn't matter— real food is exactly the same. You're going to learn skills and techniques that will immediately apply to your life, and if something doesn't fit perfectly, you can easily personalize it to make it work for you. Before you can fully embrace a real-food diet, it's important to understand what real food is.

Real food rots. As a result, real food is usually found in the refrigerator, freezer, or dried and stored in the pantry. Real food is nutritious—meaning that it contains nutritional value like carbohydrates, protein, and/or healthy fats, as well as vitamins, minerals, enzymes, and phytonutrients which are responsible for the bright colors of real foods. It's wholesome and minimally processed. It's the whole thing, not a fractionated piece, and is

REAL FOOD, REAL SIMPLE

usually a single ingredient. Real food is something that you can picture growing whether it's a plant or animal. The following categories are considered real foods:

▶ **Vegetables and leafy greens**—Vegetables come in all different colors, shapes, and sizes and are loaded with antioxidants and vitamins. Carrots, cucumbers, peppers, sweet potatoes, summer and winter squash, radishes, onions, and garlic are all examples of health-promoting vegetables. Dark leafy greens are filled with phytonutrients and minerals like calcium and iron. Lettuces (like romaine and green leaf), kale, collard greens, Swiss chard, bok choy, and spinach are all examples of leafy greens.

▶ **Fruits**—Organic, in-season fruits are filled with vitamins, minerals, phytonutrients, antioxidants, and fiber. Berries like blackberries, blueberries, raspberries, and strawberries are excellent eaten raw or tossed into smoothies. Fruit is found in most of the colors of the rainbow and includes everything from mangoes and grapes to apples and cherries.

▶ **Whole grains**—Whole grains are often cleaned and dried for storage until they are cooked. They are filled with fiber, trace minerals, vitamins, and protein. A few examples of whole grains are brown rice, whole wheat, oats, barley, and corn. Pseudo-grains like quinoa are also great choices, as they have even more protein than traditional grains and can be used interchangeably with whole grains.

▶ **Beans and legumes**—Beans and legumes include lentils; beans, like pinto beans, black beans, and garbanzo beans; as well as soy beans and soy products such as tempeh. Beans are loaded with protein, fiber, and vitamins. They are a great complement to whole grains and are a staple food in many areas of the world.

▶ **Nuts and seeds**—A great source of essential fats, protein, and minerals, nuts and seeds make a great snack or garnish. Almonds, hazelnuts, pecans, pistachios, and walnuts are all examples of nuts. Seeds include pumpkin seeds, sunflower seeds, chia seeds, flax seeds, and many others. Cold-pressed oils made from nuts and seeds are also excellent sources of essential fats. Raw nuts and seeds can actually be planted, and they will grow into a new plant given the right soil and weather conditions.

▶ **Herbs and spices**—Herbs and spices are a great addition to your real-food diet, as they provide potent phytonutrients, antioxidants, and lots of flavor. Some common herbs are parsley, cilantro, rosemary, oregano, and basil. They are found fresh amidst produce or dried in jars. Spices range from cinnamon and nutmeg to chili pepper and turmeric. Spices are often a single ingredient or prepared as a blend and sold in jars or in bulk.

▶ **Meat, poultry, and eggs**—Animal products can be a healthy addition to a real-food diet when consumed in small quantities and accompanied by lots of fresh vegetables. Look for meat, poultry, and eggs that were raised without synthetic hormones and antibiotics, and preferably grass-fed and/or organic varieties. Wild game is also a good choice, as it is leaner and contains far less saturated fat and more nutrition than farmed meat.

▶ **Seafood**—Fish and shellfish can be another healthy addition to your real-food diet. Many fish species are loaded with essential fatty acids and, when consumed at least once a week, are heart-protective and nourish your brain. Mercury contamination and sustainability are both concerns when choosing fish, so be sure to look for species low in pollutant contamination, such as wild Alaskan salmon. For more information on choosing health-promoting seafood, visit: www.gotmercury.org or www.seafoodwatch.com.

▶ **Dairy**—Dairy products like milk, butter, yogurt, and cheeses can be included in your real-food diet, if you tolerate them, for added flavor and protein. While dairy products are not appropriate for those with lactose intolerance, milk allergy, sensitivity to casein (the protein found in milk), or vegans, including dairy products is a personal choice. Dairy is a good source of calcium when accompanied by vitamin D, but don't think that dairy is the only place to get calcium. Leafy greens are an excellent source of calcium, as are sesame seeds. If you are going to include dairy products, be sure to look for organic varieties.

▶ **Water**—While it's not technically a food, water is one of the most important aspects of life and health. Pure water is used to detoxify the body by flushing out waste and toxins, nourish the cells, lubricate joints, and help the body assimilate the food you eat. Drinking at least sixty-four ounces of pure filtered water each day is essential to boost your energy and keep your body operating effectively. Water is real. Everything else is a treat for once in a while—that includes coffee, tea, juice, alcohol, soda, and anything else that you drink that's not water.

These real foods are high-quality and as close to nature as possible. They are minimally processed and usually just one ingredient. When it comes to real food, the whole is truly greater than the sum of its parts. The magic of cooking and eating happens when you start from scratch and pair up several real-food ingredients into a beautiful and nourishing home-cooked meal.

Meals made from real foods are anti-inflammatory, alkalizing, and have been proven to prevent chronic diseases like cancer and heart disease. The myriad positive health benefits of eating real food is often attributed to fresh produce like fruits, vegetables, and leafy greens as well as whole grains, nuts, and seeds.

The number one key to the incredible health benefits of real food is quality. It should be organic or as close to organic as possible. Food should be free of pesticides, growth hormones, antibiotics, heavy metals, and other toxins like PCBs and dioxin. Additionally, it should be non-GMO, or not a genetically modified organism. Meat, poultry, eggs, and dairy should be grass-fed and organic, if possible. These aspects of real food radically increase their health benefits and reduce the environmental impact of growing food.

Real food is also in season. Most Americans get fresh food from the supermarket. Grocery stores stock their produce sections and shelves with food flown in from all over the world. If you think of supermarkets as part of the global food system, where most food travels more than 2,000 miles from where it's grown to your kitchen, it's no wonder that you're probably confused about what's "in season" and what's not.

Here are some common examples of food flown in from other parts of the world: grapes from Chile, mangoes from Mexico, and pineapples from Hawaii. Asparagus doesn't grow in November in the United States; it is a spring vegetable. So if you want to buy asparagus in November, it's not going to taste nearly as good, because it was probably grown in some faraway country south of the equator and put on a plane to get to you.

Fruits and vegetables are more nutritious and delicious when they are in season. The best way to figure out what's in season in your area is to go to a farmer's market. Most farmer's markets are filled to the brim with local produce at the peak of freshness, grown in your area, and often picked just hours before you buy it. If you can't make it to a farmer's market or don't have one in your area, you can learn to navigate the supermarket for seasonal produce by checking out the Seasonal Produce Chart in Appendix A (or go to www.erinharner.com/real-food-resources/ to download the printable version) and reading labels on your food to tell you where it came from. Just be wary when shopping for produce at a grocery store. Just because it may be in season locally, doesn't mean that grocery stores actually sell the local produce.

What Real Food Is Not

"First say to yourself what you would be; and then do what you have to do." –Epictetus

Processed food has completely infiltrated our food supply. Processed food is so well adopted by Americans that our grocery stores, the place where most people buy food, are filled to the brim with aisles and aisles of food-like substances. Processed food is not real food, and it's pretty easy to spot. Food-like substances are usually found in a bag, box, or wrapper and have a nutrition-facts label on them.

Real food is not refined, polished, or processed. When food is processed in any way, it is no longer in its original, natural form. It becomes bits and pieces of the whole, and your body will crave what's missing. Here is an example: brown rice is a whole, real food. White rice is not. White rice starts out as brown rice with the bran and germ intact. Then the brown rice gets milled to remove the bran and germ, and then it's polished. The end product is white rice, which contains a lot of starch and little nutritional value.

Keep in mind that there are several levels of processing food. Wheat, for example, starts out as whole-grain wheat berries. If the wheat berries are simply ground, they make whole-wheat flour. If the wheat berries are milled to remove the bran and germ, this produces unbleached white flour. Most flour is bleached to make it even whiter, and this is the standard white flour found at the grocery store. When whole-wheat flour is made into bread, you end up with whole-wheat bread. When bleached white flour is made into bread, this is a traditional loaf of white bread. As you can see, the more processing the whole grain or whole food undergoes, the more nutritional value it loses and the less it looks like real food.

Real foods often don't have nutrition-facts labels. Think about the produce section at the grocery store. Do apples or lettuce have nutrition-facts labels? It's highly unlikely. If you're looking at a food or product that has a nutrition-facts label on it, take a look at the ingredients. Are there fewer than five ingredients? Can a seven-year-old read the ingredients? If yes, it may be a real food. If there are more than five ingredients or you wouldn't keep all of the ingredients in your kitchen cupboard, then it is not real food. If a seven-year-old couldn't read what's in it, or the first ingredient is sugar or some variation of sugar, it is not real food.

In order to make processed food more appealing and to withstand months or years of sitting on a shelf, food manufacturers use lots of different artificial flavorings, colorings, sweeteners, trans fats, and preservatives. If products have artificial sweeteners like aspartame, saccharin, or others; artificial colors like Red 40, Blue 5, or caramel coloring; artificial flavors like artificial vanilla; or preservatives other than salt, they are not good for you and definitely not real food. If the words "partially hydrogenated" are in the listed ingredients, it contains unhealthy trans fats and is not a real food. If the words "light" or "low-fat" are on the label, the manufacturer likely replaced fat with sugar or artificial sweeteners in the product. Put these items back! In addition, if a food-like product has been sugared, caffeinated, or carbonated, it is not real food. Processed foods are typically loaded with sugar, salt, and fat, and this makes them highly inflammatory when you eat them.

If a product is heavily marketed and laden with health claims, there is a very good chance that it is not real food. Food companies are competing for your food dollars, and it's really easy to get sucked into the hype. If there are health claims trying to convince you how healthy it is, be very skeptical. When is the last time you saw a commercial for carrots or broccoli? Food manufacturers pay for product positioning at the grocery store, and it works. The more processed food you buy, the more money they make. Sadly, most real foods don't have million-dollar marketing budgets. Don't get fooled, know what real food is and what it isn't.

Real food is not covered in synthetic pesticides, herbicides, or fungicides either. Real food is as close to nature as possible and is therefore organic or grown with organic practices in mind. As of 2002, USDA organic standards require that no synthetic pesticides or fertilizers are used to grow the crops. No GMOs, such as genetically modified corn, are used. Crop-rotation and soil-conservation methods are used when growing crops. Farm animals must be fed 100 percent organic feed, have access to outdoor pasture, and be administered no antibiotics or hormones.

Synthetic pesticide residues on produce are potentially toxic and a big health concern. Organic farming practices prevent synthetic pesticides from being used in growing crops. According to the Environmental Working Group, the most pesticide-contaminated produce are apples, celery, sweet bell peppers, peaches, and strawberries. Be sure to buy these fruits and vegetables organic, if you can. You can find the complete list as well as more information about pesticide residues and their health implications at www.ewg.org. If you really want to stretch your food budget and only purchase the *dirtiest* fresh vegetables and fruits as organic, you'll be making a huge upgrade to your diet and reduce the toxic burden coming into your body.

As a general rule, your calories should come from food—real food. They should not come from beverages like soda, juice (yes, even 100 percent fruit juice), sweeteners in tea or coffee, or alcohol. These products are not real food. The two exceptions are smoothies made from real food, which you end up drinking, and freshly pressed vegetable juice made from leafy greens, celery, beets, cucumbers, carrots, and other real foods—and, again, canned or bottled vegetable juices do not count.

To help you sort out what real food is versus what it is not, here are some examples:

- Apples vs. pasteurized apple juice
- Tomatoes vs. canned tomato juice
- Green beans vs. green bean chips
- Potatoes vs. fried French fries
- Brown rice vs. white rice
- Whole oats vs. instant oatmeal
- Whole grain bread vs. white bread
- Pinto beans vs. canned refried beans
- Eggs (organically produced) vs. egg whites in a carton

- Chicken breasts vs. chicken roll deli meat

- Turkey breasts vs. turkey sausage

- Plain yogurt vs. probiotic supplements

- Red grapes vs. resveratrol supplements

As shown above, supplements are not real food either. Supplements should be taken to supplement a diet filled with nutrient-dense whole real foods. Let me repeat—supplements, even the ones made from whole foods, are not real food and are certainly not a replacement for whole real food. All the supplements in the world will never make you healthy without the solid foundation of a healthy real–food diet. The purpose of supplements is to fill in the gaps of what you may be missing in your diet, or to provide enough vitamins, minerals, or another compound at a dose high enough to produce a therapeutic effect.

Supplements can significantly increase your health, and often they provide therapeutic doses of nutrients that you would be hard-pressed to get from real food, like probiotics, omega-3 fatty acids, or vitamins and minerals. These, however, are a special circumstance where your body has a specific need for additional nutrition on top of a healthy real food–based diet. When considering taking supplements, it's important to consult with a nutrition or health-care professional to help you figure out what to take, how much you need, for how long, and also to obtain high-quality supplements with potent ingredients that will have the intended effect.

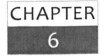

CHAPTER
6

Making the Switch to a Real-Food Diet

"A journey of a thousand miles must begin with a single step."
—Lao Tzu

Now you know what real food is and what it isn't. Transitioning from a processed-food diet to a diet filled with real foods like fresh vegetables and fruits, whole grains, and more plant-based protein takes time. It does not happen overnight, so be patient. Making the switch to a real-food diet is absolutely worth it. You'll have more energy, effortlessly lose weight until you reach your ideal weight, feel good about your body, and think a lot more clearly.

Your body is brilliant, and it wants to be healthy. If you give your body what it needs to heal itself, it will heal itself. Hippocrates, who is often referred to as the father of Western medicine, said, "Let food be thy medicine and thy medicine be thy food." Modern medicine has really gotten away from this philosophy, however. Hippocrates didn't say, "Take a pill to heal."

Real food is made up of macronutrients and micronutrients. Macronutrients are carbohydrates, proteins, and fats, and they are responsible for many of the reactions in your body, including

REAL FOOD, REAL SIMPLE

the conversion to energy. Micronutrients include vitamins, minerals, and phytonutrients. Micronutrients are essential and must come from your diet. Note that Hippocrates didn't say to "eat more protein," "take calcium supplements," or "reduce fat intake." Real food is so much greater than the sum of its parts, so focus on eating more real food and don't worry so much about all the other nutrition facts and figures like calories, fat grams, sodium content, or anything else you find on a nutrition-facts label. If you eat a diverse array of different-colored foods, different types of foods, and eat plenty of protein-rich foods, then you have nothing to worry about.

Client Story:

Dawn is a finance manager at a large company with a busy work and travel schedule. In just a few short months, Dawn went from eating a restricted diet filled with cafeteria, restaurant, and processed food to a real–food diet. She used to "feel very guilty and disgusted with [her]self all the time because [she] knew [she] was not eating healthy."

Dawn was surprised that I "insisted on eating real food, as opposed to a diet of complicated ratios of carbs, proteins, and fats." She even pointed out that in our work together "I didn't even talk about calories or grams of fat."

She is no longer eating out every night and is now cooking or preparing healthy foods at home. She's skipping vending machine raids in favor of being prepared, and brings snacks with her to work and whenever she's on the go. Also, since Dawn is a young professional who travels frequently for work, when she chooses "to go out and splurge a bit, [she] no longer feels badly about it because [she] knows that [she] is eating healthy real food most of the time."

To make a successful transition to a real food diet, start by crowding out the junk by adding in real–food. One thing you can do immediately is to quit buying processed food-like substances and start buying real food. By upgrading your choices and adding healthy whole foods into your diet, you will naturally push out the junk that's robbing your energy and getting in the way of you feeling awesome.

When you try to do something different, you'll often encounter resistance from those closest to you, whether it's your family or friends. But stick with it. They love you. Deep down, they want you to be happy and healthy, whether they show it or not. Bring something new to the family picnic. Try a new dish at dinner time, and don't apologize for it. Making real food to nourish your family, friends, or coworkers is a loving and caring thing to do. When resistance to change comes up, acknowledge it and just keep moving forward with your real food transition.

You eat three to six times each day, so making several small real-food tweaks and upgrades will add up to big changes. Start by adding in healthier staple foods, like white whole-wheat, whole-wheat, or other whole-grain bread instead of white bread, and you will encounter less resistance from family and friends and make the transition a lot easier. When you focus on making simple, healthy upgrades to the staple foods that you eat often, you will make a big impact on your diet in a short amount of time.

Making the switch to a real-food diet will force you to adopt some new habits, like preparing meals at home. You'll also need to have food in the house and a stocked kitchen to make healthy eating at home easier. Preparing meals and eating at home is critical. When you cook your own meals at home from scratch, starting with a number of fresh, single-ingredient foods that you whip up into healthy and delicious combinations, your food is prepared with love, and you have control over how it is prepared. Instead of buying food prepared by others, you can decide how much and what types of sugar, salt, and fat to add to your food. You also gain control of the quality and source of your food, and when it comes to making the transition to a real-food diet, quality is a lot more important than quantity.

To reap the enormous benefits of eating real food in a short amount of time, start with fresh produce. Fresh fruits and vegetables that are organic or grown without synthetic pesticides and herbicides are the best choice. If you have trouble making it to a grocery store or farmer's market to buy fresh produce on a weekly basis, stock up when it's in season and freeze it. Or you can buy frozen vegetables and fruits to make sure that you have vegetables and fruits in the house between shopping trips. Canned items, like canned vegetables and fruits, are the least desirable choice but can be used in a bind. Canned products are often heated, which kills some vitamins and the enzymes in the food; preserved with chemicals or salt; and stored in cans that leach.

There are a number of strategies to make eating a diet full of healthy real food work in your life, and we'll cover those in this book. For now, just realize that making the transition to a real-food diet requires a bit of creativity and a lot of perseverance. Just keep at it and get support from a nutrition coach, friend, or family member if you need it.

Conquering Cravings

Cravings for different types of foods are pretty common when you're eating a highly processed diet, and they are a sign that your body gives you when something isn't quite right. Understanding what cravings mean and how to deal with them will help you make a smooth transition from a diet filled with processed food to a nutrient-dense real-food diet.

When you eat more real foods, you'll start to notice that you have fewer cravings for sweet or salty foods and your mood will stabilize as well. Instead of major swings from sweet to salty and salty to sweet that often occur as a result of low energy or consuming lots of processed foods and caffeine, you will get off the blood-sugar roller coaster and start to feel more calm and confident.

One of the reasons that cravings occur when you're eating a heavily processed diet is that processed food is simply fractionated bits of what was formerly food, and your body notices that something is missing. If you find that you're craving a lot of sweet foods, try eating more fruit; add in sweet vegetables like sweet potatoes, carrots, or beets; and use natural sweeteners like stevia. If you notice that you frequently crave salty foods, try drinking more water and eating fewer sweet foods. This will naturally help your body balance out.

Also, because processed food is largely devoid of nutrition, it keeps you hungry and wanting more. When you eat junk, your body wants more and more food and is never truly satisfied because the food is empty—you're eating, but your body isn't getting what it's looking for from the food. Your body is fed, but it's not nourished. When you eat real food, your body will start to tell you when you're done. Because the food you're eating is full of nutrition, it stops wanting more and more food to fill the void. You'll find yourself eating less and feeling more satisfied.

You will also notice, when you transition to a nutrient-dense real-food diet, that your cravings for certain foods that you thought you couldn't live without just go away. It won't take long, and in fact, for most of my clients, it takes only a few days for their bodies to get rid of the toxic junk coming into them from their over-processed diets and to stop craving foods that they really don't want anyway.

Client Story:

Cheryl is a physician who was struggling with low energy, poor digestion, and insatiable cravings for fast food and chips. Despite having a good idea about what she should be eating, Cheryl was overwhelmed by the thought of cooking healthy meals and instead chose to eat out frequently.

After I worked with Cheryl for a couple months, she noticed incredible improvements in her energy, digestion, and cravings. She is now shopping for healthy food and cooking meals each week. She no longer has cravings for chips and fast food and knows how to conquer her cravings when she starts craving foods that aren't "real food." By switching to a real food diet and ditching the junk, Cheryl even lost seven pounds in two months without trying. Now that's pretty cool.

Healthy Eating on a Budget

When you transition to a diet full of nutrient-dense foods, you will undoubtedly pay more money for food. Our highly processed food supply is filled with cheap food and every imaginable combination of corn, soy, and wheat, which are subsidized by the government to make them artificially inexpensive.

Sadly, an organic apple may cost more than a fast-food cheeseburger. That is the up-front cost, however. If you think about the nutritional value in each, it's not hard to realize that the apple is actually a much better deal, as it is filled with vitamins, minerals, enzymes, fiber, and natural sugars that will actually give you energy. The fast-food hamburger is filled with a small percentage of low-quality meat, meat fillers, lots of salt, likely some mystery ingredients like preservatives or monosodium glutamate (MSG), and then it's fried in oil that may or may not contain trans fats. And that is just the burger! When you add in the bleached-white-flour bun and slice of processed cheese food, you've got a "cheeseburger" of very little nutritional value that is going to make you tired instead of giving you energy like food should.

Paying a bit more for high-quality food up front will very likely end up saving you a lot of money later, whether it's on doctor bills, prescription medications, high-cost treatments for chronic diseases, and so on. So if you find yourself or others griping about the higher cost of high-quality nutrient-dense food, think about the long-term costs associated with low-quality food and make a choice.

As you branch out and start eating more high-quality real food, your grocery bill will go up, but there are ways to shop smart and plan what you're going to eat to minimize a spike in your monthly food bill. In the next several chapters, we'll discuss how to set up your real-food kitchen and make healthy cooking and eating easier as a result of having pantry staples and core foods that you eat often in the house. This will save you time and money, since you'll be shopping for food less and cooking at home more. We'll also discuss which kitchen tools, utensils, and appliances will make your life easier. By having these in your home and learning some basic cutting techniques, meal-preparation techniques, and cooking techniques, you will be better equipped to cut and prepare ingredients at home. As a result, you'll be buying bags of large carrots instead of baby carrots and chopping them yourself. You could buy a fresh pineapple and slice it, for example, instead of buying cans of pineapple chunks or cut pineapple at the grocery store or market, which will also save you money.

Eating healthy on a budget also becomes a lot easier when you learn how to plan meals ahead of time, shop for and purchase only what you actually need for the week, and prevent food spoilage because you don't have extra food that is not on your meal plan hanging around waiting to be eaten.

Another simple way to save money and prevent your food bill from getting out of control when making the transition to a healthier real-food diet is to emphasize vegetarian sources of protein, like lentils, beans, or eggs, which are much less expensive than high-quality fish, poultry, or meat. When you combine lentils or beans with whole grains that complement them, like brown rice, you can create healthy, delicious, and complete meals for less. Remember to emphasize quality over quantity. So if grass-fed, free-range, or organic animal products will only fit into your budget once or twice a week, instead of compromising the quality of the food, just choose another option, as there are lots of great inexpensive protein sources out there.

Additionally, because you'll be cooking a lot more at home and eating out less, you will save money on your meals. High-quality real-food meals at home are almost always less expensive than eating out, so keep that in mind as well as you continue reading and implementing the tips and strategies in this book.

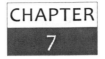

Setting Up Your Real-Food Kitchen

"There are no shortcuts to any place worth going." –Beverly Sills

Healthy eating works when you create an environment that supports it. It's critical to make sure that you have what you need in your kitchen to make healthy meals fast. Having healthy ingredients on hand as well as essential kitchen tools, utensils, and appliances makes preparing healthy meals much easier.

Start by taking an inventory of your kitchen. Look through your pantry, cupboards, refrigerator, and freezer and ask, "Is this real food?" If it's not real food, get rid of it. Donate it to your local food pantry, compost it, or throw it away. Take some time to create a blank slate. Decluttering and getting rid of the processed food-like substances makes cooking and eating healthy infinitely easier, so do not skip this step! When your kitchen is filled with real food, you will create an environment in your home that fully supports a healthy real-food diet.

A big key to consistently eating a healthy real-food diet is to make healthy eating the obvious and only choice. Your home is a controlled environment where you or your family members bring food into the house. Ask for support from your family and friends to only bring real food into your house. This is easier said than done, but keep in mind that you have complete control over what comes in the front door. To create an environment in your home that supports your health goals and makes you feel really good, don't let junk food enter. Only bring real food into your home, and it will become the only and obvious choice of what to eat.

Preparing healthy meals in thirty minutes or less is a breeze when you have real food in your kitchen and the right tools, kitchen utensils, and appliances. Let's dig into the stuff that belongs in your kitchen.

The Food

There are several foods that are helpful to keep on hand in your real-food kitchen. As you go through your pantry, cupboards, refrigerator, and freezer, discard all foods that are old, rancid, or considered junk. Here are the real-food staples to start stocking your kitchen with. You probably won't have some of the real-food items on this list in your kitchen currently, and that is okay. As you cook an increasing variety of real-food meals and increase your recipe repertoire, slowly add in new pantry and perishable staples.

▶ **Vegetables and leafy greens:** Seasonal vegetables are fresh and at the peak of ripeness and nutrition. Look for organic and local vegetables like carrots, celery, leafy greens (like kale, Swiss chard, lettuce, and spinach), broccoli, tomatoes, summer and winter squash, sweet potatoes, beets, and cauliflower. Also keep onions, garlic, and fresh ginger on hand year-round for use in many savory dishes. When some vegetables are not in season, keep organic frozen corn, peas, and spinach in the freezer to add variety to your real-food diet. Cultured vegetables and raw sauerkraut are great to keep in the refrigerator to eat with meals or as a snack. Tomatoes are great to keep in the pantry as diced or crushed canned tomatoes, sun-dried tomatoes, and tomato paste. Green and black olives, capers, and pickles in jars keep well in the pantry until opened and are tasty additions to meals. Vegetable broth is great to have for soups and to add extra flavor to whole grains as they are cooking. Also, look for sea vegetables like dulse flakes, kelp, kombu, and wakame to add flavor and minerals to meals, or use nori sheets as an edible wrapper.

▶ **Fruits:** Fresh fruits are seasonal, so choose fruit that is ripe, fresh, and preferably local. Look for apples, pears, blueberries, strawberries, cherries, melon, grapefruit, oranges, lemons, and other fruit when it's in season. Berries like blueberries, strawberries, blackberries, and raspberries; bananas; mangoes; and other fruits freeze for well when they are not in season. Keep these fruits in your freezer for smoothies, fruit sauces, and other fruit treats. Dried fruit is versatile and keeps well. Try raisins, apricots, cranberries, cherries, and apples. Store dried fruit in glass jars in the pantry to keep it fresh. Jam is notoriously high in sugar, so look for unsweetened apple butter and fruit spreads with no added sugar or fruit spreads sweetened with fruit juice instead.

▶ **Whole grains:** Whole grains should be used up or replaced every six months and kept in airtight containers, like glass jars, in a cool, dark place. Look for organic varieties of quinoa (white and red), millet, buckwheat or kasha (roasted buckwheat), Arborio rice, short- or medium-grain brown rice, and brown basmati rice. Also look for thick rolled oats, steel-cut oats, corn meal, popcorn kernels, and whole-wheat flour. If you're gluten-free, look for brown-rice flour, sorghum flour, quinoa flour, buckwheat flour, tapioca starch, and any other gluten-free whole-grain flour that you enjoy.

▶ **Whole-grain products:** It's helpful to keep some products made from whole grains in your kitchen for when you need to put together a quick meal. Cold cereals like oat bran, granola, and raw muesli are great for breakfast or as toppings for yogurt or dessert. Soba noodles and whole-wheat pasta are great as well for a quick dinner. Sprouted whole-grain bread, whole-wheat pitas, and corn tortillas are also convenient to keep on hand. You can freeze them for later use if you use them rarely. If you're gluten-free, look for brown-rice pasta, quinoa pasta, and brown-rice tortillas to make wraps.

▶ **Beans and legumes:** In order to cook properly, beans need to be fresh, so store them in glass jars in a cool, dark place and use them up or replace them every six months. Look for organic varieties of dried kidney beans, black beans, pinto beans, garbanzo beans, split peas, and lentils. If you're transitioning to a real-food diet and are not used to planning meals or cooking from scratch, keep a few cans of organic and salt-free kidney beans, black beans, pinto beans, white beans, and garbanzo beans in your pantry for when you don't have time to soak and cook dried beans. In addition, organic tempeh and tofu can be kept in the fridge for occasional use in dishes.

▶ **Meat, poultry, and seafood:** Meat and poultry should be raised without antibiotics and hormones and should also be free-range or organic, if possible. Look for chicken, turkey, and lean beef or bison. Beef broth and free-range chicken broth can be kept in the pantry and are useful to add flavor to dishes. Fish and seafood can be a healthy part of a real-food diet. Choose sustainably harvested seafood with low heavy-metal contamination, like wild Alaskan salmon, wild cod, scallops, or tilapia. Sardines, tuna in water, and boneless and skinless salmon in water can also be convenient occasional additions, as they keep well.

▶ **Dairy products and eggs:** If you consume dairy, look for organic milk, butter, cheeses, and Greek or plain yogurt. If you're dairy-free, look for unsweetened varieties of hemp milk, rice milk, or almond milk. Coconut milk is essential for some curries and gives other dairy-free dishes a creamy texture. Look for organic or free-range, antibiotic- and hormone-free eggs.

▶ **Nuts and seeds:** Look for raw nuts and seeds in the bulk section of many stores. Store raw nuts and seeds in glass jars in the freezer to keep them fresh. Walnuts, almonds, cashews, pine nuts, sunflower seeds, pumpkin seeds, sesame seeds, flaxseeds, and chia seeds will meet most of your culinary needs. Nut and seed butters have many uses and should be natural and organic, if possible. Store them in the refrigerator once opened to keep them fresh. Look for unsalted natural peanut butter, almond butter, cashew butter, tahini (ground sesame seed butter), and sunflower seed butter.

▶ **Oils:** You don't need many oils. A few high-quality unrefined oils will meet all of your cooking and baking needs. Try to find organic oils and store them in a cool, dark place to prevent them from going rancid. Stock your pantry with extra-virgin olive oil for salad dressings, dips, and spreads or low-temperature sautéing; flaxseed oil for salad dressings;

virgin coconut oil and grapeseed oil for medium- to high-temperature cooking and baking; and toasted sesame oil and hot-pepper sesame oil as a garnish for stir-fries, sauces, marinades, and leafy greens.

▶ **Vinegars and cooking wines:** Use vinegars and cooking wines at the end of cooking as a garnish to enhance the flavor. Look for organic varieties and store in a cool, dark place to keep them fresh. Apple cider vinegar, balsamic vinegar, brown-rice vinegar, red and white wine vinegar, and umeboshi or ume plum vinegar (salty and sour) are all highly versatile. Sherry, sherry vinegar, and cooking wine also enhance the natural flavor or dishes.

▶ **Natural sweeteners:** Refined sweeteners like white and brown sugar have been stripped of nutrients like vitamins and minerals that help to metabolize the sugar. Natural sweeteners are less processed and maintain most of their original nutritional value. Use them whenever refined sugars are called for in recipes. Look for pure maple syrup, raw honey, Medjool dates, brown rice syrup, coconut palm sugar, agave nectar, blackstrap molasses, and stevia extract.

▶ **Herbs and spices:** These give an array of flavors and colors to food. Replace ground spices and herbs annually to ensure that they are fresh and flavorful. Keep dried spices on hand like cinnamon, ginger, cumin, cardamom, cayenne pepper, paprika, turmeric, ground black pepper, garlic powder, mustard seed, and blends like chili powder, curry powder, and garam masala. Dried herbs like parsley, basil, oregano, thyme, rosemary, and bay leaves are versatile and add flavor and color when fresh herbs aren't available. Dried spices and herbs only stay fresh and potent for six to twelve months so date them when you buy them. Fresh herbs like basil, mint, cilantro, and parsley store for several days in the refrigerator and are immensely useful in cooking fresh, flavorful, and nutritious dishes.

▸ **Salt and salt substitutes:** Salt brings out the natural flavor of dishes when used in small quantities. Look for Celtic sea salt to use for cooking and baking. A salt mill is helpful for grinding coarse salt crystals. Bragg's Liquid Aminos, organic seasoned salt, and a sea salt and sesame seed combination called gomasio all make great substitutions for pure salt. Traditional soy sauce (made from wheat and soy) and tamari (gluten-free soy sauce) are also great salt substitutes and impart their own flavor.

▸ **Condiments and other kitchen staples:** Other toppings like naturally sweetened ketchup, Dijon mustard, miso paste, wasabi, hot chili sauce, and horseradish give certain dishes a flavor boost. Dips and spreads like hummus, baba ghanoush, and salsa are great for dipping vegetables. Nutritional yeast is a great popcorn topper and supplies loads of B vitamins. Vanilla extract and raw cacao or cocoa powder are versatile kitchen staples that add flavor to smoothies and desserts.

▸ **Tea:** Green tea and herbal teas are great to keep on hand for making hot tea and iced teas as well.

For a complete list of recommended staples for your real-food kitchen, download the Real Food Kitchen Staples Checklist at www.erinharner.com/real-food-resources/.

The Kitchen Essentials

Kitchen tools, utensils, and appliances in working order are must-haves for your real-food kitchen in order to cook healthy meals efficiently. As you start to cook more and more, you'll learn which kitchen tools and appliances make your life easier and which ones you can do without. When it comes to kitchen tools, quality is much more important than quantity. We'll start with the must-have kitchen tools, utensils, and appliances.

▶ **Bakeware:** Most bakeware is either metal or glass. Dark metal and glass baking dishes hold more heat and cook faster than shiny metal bakeware, so use whichever works best for you. The essential bakeware for your kitchen includes an eight- or nine-inch pie plate, a loaf pan for quick breads, 9" x 13" baking dishes, and cookie sheets with raised sides.

▶ **Blender:** A blender with a glass pitcher will last longer and is more adaptable for puréeing soups or smoothies. An immersion blender is a handheld blender wand that you can insert into pots or glasses to blend smoothies or soups. Choose the type of blender that best meets your needs; you don't necessarily need both.

▶ **Can opener:** Essential for opening cans of beans, tomatoes, black olives, or other foods. A small metal can opener with rubber or plastic grips on the handles is all you need to open cans with little effort.

▶ **Colander/strainer:** A large metal colander with medium holes is helpful to strain pasta or rinse fruit. A medium-size (about seven inches across) fine mesh strainer is essential for rinsing beans, lentils, and grains or straining liquids.

▶ **Cutting boards:** There are many different types of cutting boards, including wood, bamboo, and plastic. Plastic cutting boards are light and easy to clean but tend to dull knives faster than wood or bamboo. They also wear faster than wood or bamboo with use. Wood or bamboo cutting boards last longer and don't dull knives, but they are heavier, more bulky, and harder to clean. Choose whichever cutting boards you prefer, but make sure that you have at least one large and a couple medium cutting boards. That way, you can have a designated cutting board for meat, poultry, and seafood, another for onions and garlic, and another for fruit, vegetables, and everything else.

▶ **Glass food storage bowls:** Leftover foods should be stored in the refrigerator in glass bowls. A variety of sizes are helpful for different quantities of ingredients. Be sure to get the kind with washable lids to keep food fresh and prevent lots of plastic-wrap waste.

▶ **Graters:** A box grater has four sides with different blades for grating cheeses or vegetables. A microplane grater or zester has a handle and either a course or fine blade. Microplane graters make grating spices like nutmeg or fresh ginger, zesting lemons or limes, and finely grating cheeses simple.

▶ **Knives:** Perhaps the most useful kitchen tool, you only need a few high-quality sharp knives to cut just about everything in the kitchen. There are stainless steel, ceramic, and carbon steel knives on the market, each with their own advantages. Use whichever type you prefer, but three to four sharp stainless steel knives will be more than sufficient to get you started. Look for full tang-knives, where the blade extends all the way through the handle. Choose whichever knives suit the majority of your kitchen needs. Here are some excellent options: paring knife for peeling fruits and vegetables; six, eight, or ten inch chef's knife for slicing and chopping; cleaver for slicing thick-skinned winter vegetables; and a small or large serrated knife for slicing bread or tomatoes.

❱ **Lunch and travel containers:** Containers to take food with you make healthy eating easy when you're on the go. Many lunch or travel containers are plastic with locking lids. Stainless steel interlocking containers are also great to use, last a long time, and are easy to clean.

❱ **Measuring cups and spoons:** Glass measuring cups (two- and four-cup capacity) are helpful for measuring liquid ingredients. Stainless steel measuring cups are great for dry ingredients like flours because you can scrape excess off the top. Stainless steel measuring spoons are often found on a ring, are easy to clean, and are used for measuring small amounts of wet or dry ingredients.

❱ **Mixing bowls:** Glass and/or stainless steel mixing bowls are highly adaptable for a variety of uses, including mixing ingredients, preparing food, serving, or even storing foods in glass bowls with lids. Look for glass or stainless steel mixing bowls that stack to save space in your cupboards.

❱ **Pots and pans:** The pots and pans that will be useful for you depend on how many people you typically cook for. If you're cooking for one or two, you'll need smaller pots and pans than if you have a family of six or do a lot of canning, freezing, or food preservation yourself. In general, high-quality stainless steel pots and pans in assorted sizes and volumes will be helpful. A two-quart saucepan is one of the most versatile pots in your kitchen, as you can use it for cooking grains, sautéing vegetables, or making sauces. A stock pot is great for making soups, stews, or pasta and usually comes in a six- or twelve-quart size. A sauté pan that is ten or twelve inches in diameter is useful for sautéing meat or vegetables. A larger sauté pan is great for cooking greens, making chili, or a variety of one-dish meals. Look for a four- to six-quart sauté pan with straight sides, two handles for lifting, and a lid. The final everyday pot or pan is a small, six- to seven-inch skillet used for cooking eggs, toasting nuts, or cooking small quantities of ingredients. Avoid nonstick pans coated with Teflon.

▶ **Spatulas:** Rubber spatulas are great to help with scraping and spreading. Heat-resistant flat plastic spatulas or flat metal spatulas are great for flipping pancakes on the stove, flipping meat on the grill, or removing cookies from a cookie sheet.

▶ **Spoons:** Wooden spoons are great for stirring dishes on the stove as well as serving. A variety of wooden spoons, including solid, slotted, and flat-bottomed, will meet most of your stirring, mixing, and serving needs. Metal serving spoons and a ladle for soups or stews are also helpful tools for your kitchen.

▶ **Storage jars and containers:** Pint-, quart-, and gallon-sized glass jars with either plastic lids or metal foodsafe lids are extremely useful for storing food and keeping it fresh. Dried beans, whole grains, nuts, seeds, dried fruit, and other real food is best stored in airtight glass containers. Some plastic storage containers can be helpful for freezing leftover meals, cooked whole grains, and cooked beans, if your glass storage containers are not freezer safe. Glass jars with straight sides and plastic lids usually freeze well and keep soups, stews, nuts, and seeds fresh in the freezer until you're ready to use them.

▶ **Tongs:** They are great for flipping foods on the grill, serving salads or hard-to-grab foods, or turning foods in a pan on the stove. Tongs with a spring-loaded hinge are especially useful.

▶ **Vegetable peeler:** A simple vegetable peeler is helpful for peeling carrots, cucumbers, potatoes, and a number of other foods.

Other kitchen tools are not essential but may make your life simpler. These are nice to have when you need them and will make certain tasks faster and easier. If you have no use for something, don't buy it or keep it in your kitchen just in case you need it once a year—that is a waste of money and valuable kitchen space. Only keep these items in your kitchen if they will help you out.

▶ **Apple peeler:** This handy device peels, cores, and pits apples. It's helpful in the fall when apples are ripe to prepare them for dehydration, apple pies, crisps, cobblers, and applesauce.

▶ **Citrus juicer:** A citrus juicer with a dish to collect the juice or a hand citrus reamer is great for juicing lemons and oranges.

▶ **Cookie scoop:** A teaspoon- or tablespoon-size cookie scoop helps you make uniform cookies and also makes short work of other round-shaped foods like meatballs, falafel, and desserts.

▶ **Dehydrator:** Whether you want to dry herbs, fruits, or vegetables; make jerky; or dehydrate raw baked goods like kale chips, a dehydrator can be a helpful kitchen tool. Look for one with a variable temperature setting and square trays. Dehydrators are large and require a lot of kitchen storage space, so make sure you really need it before you invest in one.

▶ **Dutch oven:** A versatile pot that can go from oven to stovetop, a Dutch oven is great for one-pot meals, as it can function as a slow cooker, sauce pot, pudding pot, or baking dish. Look for a high-quality Dutch oven, and it will last a lifetime.

▶ **Electric mixer:** A small handheld electric mixer or a larger stand-up mixer is helpful for mixing dough, batters, or whipping other foods. Look for an electric mixer with multiple attachments to increase its versatility.

▶ **Food processor:** A high-quality food processor is a helpful addition to your real-food kitchen as you make more vegetable and fruit dishes. It makes shredding, slicing, and chopping foods very easy and often much faster than you could do by hand. You can also use a food processor for puréeing foods like dips, hummus, or frozen-fruit desserts. Food processors often take up a lot of storage space and have several parts to clean, so make sure you really need it before you invest in one.

▶ **Garlic press:** Once you peel garlic and remove the skins, put whole cloves in a garlic press to crush for recipes. Look for a sturdy stainless steel garlic press that is easy to clean.

▶ **High-powered blender:** A regular blender works, however a high-powered blender like the Vitamix has some noteworthy features due to its high-powered motor. Depending on the blades or canister that you use, high-powered blenders make short work of puréeing soups, smoothies, frozen fruit, and ice. They can also grind nuts into fresh nut butters or nut flours, and whole grains into flours.

▶ **Juicer:** Juicing vegetables, fruits, and herbs is a great way to get lots of high-quality nutrition into your diet without having to prepare, cook, and eat the same quantity of produce. Because juice is raw, it preserves the vitamins, minerals, and enzymes in the produce as well. Juicers are really good at juicing produce but tend to be large, heavy, and somewhat tedious to clean, so be sure you really need one before you invest. If you have a high-powered blender, you can make juice in it and simply strain it through a fine mesh strainer or cheesecloth, which would eliminate the need for a juicer.

▶ **Pressure cooker:** If you cook beans, a pressure cooker is really helpful. Because the pot is sealed and food cooks at high temperatures in a pressure cooker, foods like beans cook much faster, retain more vitamins and minerals, and are easier to digest when compared with conventional cooking.

▶ **Rice cooker:** A rice cooker can be used to cook rice or other grains and often comes with a steaming basket to steam vegetables at the same time. Rice cookers make cooking rice easy, as all you have to do is push a button, and when it's done cooking, it will switch settings to "warm" until you're ready to eat it.

▶ **Salad spinner:** After you wash salad greens or herbs, a salad spinner is helpful for drying them.

▶ **Slow cooker:** A slow cooker is a worthwhile investment if you're busy and away from home often. It allows you to cook simple meals while you're away and time them so your food is ready when you come home. Look for a slow cooker with variable heat settings and a built-in timer.

▶ **Thermometer:** To check if meat or poultry are cooked through, use a thermometer to check their internal temperature.

▶ **Vegetable-steaming basket:** A metal basket that expands and collapses to fit into most pots, a vegetable-steaming basket makes steaming fresh vegetables easy.

▶ **Whisks:** Hand whisks are usually stainless steel or coated with heat-resistant silicone. They are useful for whipping up batters by hand, beating eggs, or stirring dishes like puddings on the stove.

▶ **Wok:** Many Asian dishes like stir-fry are best cooked in a wok. The tall sloping sides allow you to easily toss the vegetables and other ingredients in the wok while they are cooking.

For a complete list of the recommended tools for your real-food kitchen, download the Real Food Kitchen Tools Checklist at www.erinharner.com/real-food-resources/.

A meal-planning binder is another really helpful tool to make preparing healthy real-food meals simple. The only requirement is that it works for you, so personalize it and make it fit the way you think and work. It should include meal-planning worksheets, a list of your favorite meals and snacks, recipes for all of your favorite meals and snacks, and recipes for dishes you'd like to try or dishes you like to make for special occasions. Your meal-planning binder is also a great place to keep recipes you find online or those given to you by friends or family. The great thing about a meal-planning binder is that it makes meal planning and cooking really simple, as everything you need is all in one place.

Cookbooks are another helpful tool for your real-food kitchen. They are great for inspiring you to try something new. When you

REAL FOOD, REAL SIMPLE

bring a new ingredient home or don't know how to make a dish you'd like to try, they are a great place to start to find a recipe. The key with cookbooks is to make sure that the ones you are using have healthy real-food recipes in them. If your cookbooks aren't filled to the brim with healthy real-food recipes, go online to find recipes, or treat yourself to a new cookbook or two that have healthy real-food recipes in them (see appendix D for cookbook recommendations). You can even copy recipes from cookbooks for your personal use and add them to your meal-planning binder so all of your favorite recipes are in one place for easy reference when you're meal planning or preparing food.

Getting Real-Food Meals on the Table

"Failing to plan is planning to fail." –Alan Lakein

You have a lot of different obligations, and getting healthy meals on the table is just one of them. It is counterintuitive, but the busier you are, the more important it is to plan ahead. Simply having a plan to eat healthy real-food meals every day of the week will also make a huge difference in your motivation and desire to actually make it happen.

Unlike popular cooking shows that make whipping up gourmet meals look easy, you don't have a sous-chef hiding out in the wings planning and prepping all of your ingredients for you. Julia Child once said, "You don't have to cook fancy or complicated masterpieces—just good food from fresh ingredients." You have a kitchen to prepare healthy meals, and they don't have to be gourmet; they just need to be fast and healthy.

Now that your kitchen is fully stocked with the food and the kitchen appliances, utensils, and tools to make food preparation and cooking easier, you're ready to get healthy meals on the table. Eating healthy does not happen by chance, accident, or some stroke of fate—it must be planned! There are four main aspects of getting healthy meals on the table, and in this chapter you'll learn how to plan meals ahead of time, shop for fresh real food, store fresh food and prevent it from spoiling, as well as critical tools and techniques to prepare healthy and delicious meals from scratch quickly and effectively. Let's jump in and make it happen.

Meal Planning

Meal planning eliminates the guesswork at mealtimes and gets rid of the "I don't know what's for dinner, let's get takeout" and "Want to order a pizza?" nights. If the words "meal planning" conjures up scary images of you sitting at the kitchen table for hours looking through cookbooks each week, don't worry. Meal planning is incredibly simple once you get the hang of it. After you create weekly meal plans for a couple weeks, you'll know exactly what to do, and it should only take about five minutes.

Creating weekly meal plans seems to be most effective, but if you live in a rural location or only shop for food every other week, creating a meal plan for two weeks at a time will be more effective so you can get what you need for both weeks at once. Be sure that you create your meal plan for the week before you go shopping. Also, you may only want to plan dinners because you take dinner leftovers for lunch the next day. You could also plan breakfast and lunch if you frequently make something different for breakfast and lunch. It's up to you—meal planning is personal. Create a system that works for you.

In chapter seven, you learned how to create a meal-planning binder. It's a really helpful tool to use to make meal planning simple. Your binder should contain meal-planning worksheets (go to www.erinharner.com/real-food-resources/ to download the Meal-Planning Worksheet), a list of your favorite meals and snacks, and recipes for your favorite meals as well as recipes for special occasions. The binder serves as your "cheat sheet" to make meal planning easy, since everything you need is all in one place. If you cook for a partner and/or kids, ask them to make a list of their favorite meals and snacks so you can incorporate those into your meal plan each week. Keep these "favorites lists" in your meal-planning binder and upgrade the recipes or meals where necessary to real-food ingredients.

Most families eat about twenty meals per week regularly, so use your upgraded meals and snacks list and your favorite-meals lists as a recipe bank to plug meals into your meal-planning worksheet. If you haven't already printed off a meal-planning worksheet, do that now. Let's get meal planning with a simple four-step process!

The first question to ask is, "Are there any events, birthdays, or holidays this week that affect meals?" Next, "Do I have anything that needs to be used up?" Look in your refrigerator and pantry and take an inventory of what you already have. If anything needs to be used up before it goes bad, write it down and be sure to incorporate it into your meal plan for the week. When you're planning meals, always start in the fridge with fresh produce.

Next, fill out the meals-for-the-week chart with what you're going to prepare for each meal. When planning meals, aim to fill half of each plate with vegetables, one quarter with protein-rich foods like meat, fish, poultry, eggs or beans, and one quarter with carbohydrate-rich foods like whole grains, root vegetables, or fruit. To make sure that you're making enough food and not too much food for your meals, you can use the hand analogy to estimate serving sizes. A serving of vegetables fits into two open hands and is about a cup; a serving of whole grains, starchy vegetables, or fruit is about half a cup or the size of your closed fist; a serving of protein-rich foods like lean meat, poultry, seafood, eggs, or beans is about three ounces or the size of your open palm; and, a serving of nuts, seeds, nut butter, fat, oil, or guacamole is one to two tablespoons or the size of your thumb. Memorizing the hand analogy will also help you buy enough ingredients for your meals each week. Use the Real Food Meals Chart (download it at www.erinharner.com/real-food-resources/) to help you plan healthy, balanced meals with lots of produce.

If you anticipate leftovers, include them in the meal plan so they don't go to waste. Also, if there is any prep that is needed to make the meals quickly, include that where appropriate. For example, brown rice should be soaked for at least eight hours. So if you're going to have brown rice for dinner one night, make a note to soak it starting the night before. That way, it's soaked and ready to go when you're ready to make dinner. If you're not going to be home until late one night, either plan to make a really quick meal for that night, plan to have leftovers, or make it ahead.

As you are filling out the meals for the week in the chart, think about any weekly meal traditions you may have already, or consider starting some. For example, if Friday night is pizza night, instead of ordering takeout pizza or going out for pizza, consider starting a make-your-own pizza night each Friday, where the whole family participates in making the pizza and putting their favorite toppings on it. Another idea is to have each family member choose a night each week for their choice of meal. This gets the whole family on board with choosing meals and helping out with meal planning. Something else you can try that works really well to make meal planning simple is to designate a cuisine for each night of the week. For example, you could have Mexican Mondays, Italian Tuesdays, Indian Wednesdays, Thai Thursdays, and so on. However you plan out your meal plan is entirely up to you and your family. Just find a way to make it work. If you'd like some help getting started, check out the Sample Real-Food Meal Plans for summer and winter in appendix B or print them out online at www.erinharner.com/real-food-resources/.

The final step involved in making your real-food meal plan is to take a look at the meals and recipes you chose for the week and make sure that you have all of the ingredients. If you don't have something, write it on your shopping list. If you're cooking

Client Story:

Liz is a research coordinator at a hospital and constantly on the go. Before we worked together, she "was having trouble figuring out what to eat in this crazy nutrition world" and struggling with the "practical aspects of getting healthy meals on the table." She was "eating out a ton because she didn't have a meal plan and felt overwhelmed with the thought of grocery shopping and cooking every single night." When Liz learned my simple meal-planning process, she was hooked.

Liz started taking thirty minutes on the weekend to plan all of her meals for the week and now she goes grocery shopping for what she needs. She is "making healthy meals every night quickly" and also making larger portions of food to take for lunch the next day. She is no longer eating the same things every single week either. Instead, she's trying new foods and asks, "What is the worst that can happen? You may not like pineapple or Swiss chard."

for one or cooking for four or more, it's important to consider how much of each ingredient you'll need for your recipes. When you're writing ingredients and amounts on your shopping list, decide whether you're planning to halve the recipe, double the recipe, or intentionally make leftovers to use in another meal, freeze, or take for lunch the next day. This will keep your fridge, freezer, and pantry stocked with all the real-food ingredients that you need to make healthy meals every day of the week.

Shopping

Food shopping ensures that you have what you need in your kitchen to make healthy real-food meals. When you shop for groceries with a list of food you actually need (because it's on your meal plan), you'll eliminate a lot of wasted food and save a ton of money. Whenever you go shopping, always take your list and try to stick to what's on it.

When you're shopping for fresh produce, look for local and organic items first. Fruits, vegetables, and herbs should look fresh and vibrant. If it is damaged, decaying, wilting, or overripe, don't buy it. Produce that is fresh, ripe, and in season is full of flavor and nutrition and will also enhance your transition to a real-food diet because it tastes delicious and you'll want to eat more of it.

There are lots of different venues to buy food, and each has its perks. You can shop for fresh local produce at local farmer's markets. Many farmer's markets only allow vendors to sell food produced within a certain radius from the market, like thirty or a hundred miles. This ensures that the food sold there is local and in season. Many farms that sell at farmer's markets are also organic, and the freshness can't be beat since the food is often picked the day before or the day of the market. When certain fruits or vegetables are ripe, in season, and plentiful, it's a good time to buy them because they are at their peak and are usually much less expensive.

CSA or Community Supported Agriculture is a growing farm-to-consumer movement where shoppers buy a share of the farm's produce. Many farm shares are all vegetables, but some farms have fruit, egg, cheese, meat, or bread shares as well. If you're looking for a consistent supply of fresh local produce and other real-food products during the growing season, a CSA is a great investment and will likely save you hundreds of dollars over the course of the summer and fall. Many CSAs also have winter shares to supply you with root vegetables and hearty leafy greens throughout the winter, depending on where you live.

Aside from farmer's markets and CSAs, health-food stores and food co-ops are often the next-best place to find fresh local and/or organic produce. They also supply specialty items that might be hard to find in regular grocery stores. Health food stores and food co-ops are also great for buying pantry staples in bulk, like beans, nuts, seeds, whole grains, dried fruit, and others. These stores are usually smaller than grocery stores and have lower product turnover, therefore they tend to be a bit more expensive for some items, but not always.

Grocery stores are where most Americans buy their food. The biggest challenge of shopping for real food at grocery stores is that they are filled with processed food-like substances backed by health claims and million-dollar marketing campaigns. In short, it's incredibly easy to get distracted when you shop at supermarkets and to veer from your shopping list. Grocery stores are best for general items like canned beans, frozen vegetables, dairy products, whole-grain products, canned tomatoes, condiments, paper towels, and napkins. Try to stay on the perimeter of the store and only go down aisles that have items on your list.

Another place to buy food is through online retailers like www. amazon.com and specialty companies like www.nuts.com that have items in bulk that may be hard to find at a location near you. One word of caution when shopping online for food is to pay close attention to the quality of the food. If it's highly processed, easy to stock for months or years, and people want it, online retailers will stock it. If you buy food online, try to stick to real-food bulk items like nuts, seeds, and specialty flours.

Remember when you're shopping to look for items that don't have nutrition-facts panels first, like fruits, vegetables, and leafy greens. Also look for bulk items like nuts, seeds, dried fruit, whole grains, and whole-grain flours. When you're shopping and trying to decide if something is a real food or not, check the nutrition-facts label, if it has one, and the ingredients list.

Read the ingredients list first, because the majority of what's in the product will be in there, but you may need to do some detective work. Ingredients are listed by quantity (weight) on the label, so start at the top. If sugar or anything that looks like sugar or ends in "–ose" is in the first three ingredients, it's packed with added sugar and definitely not a real food. If the words "partially hydrogenated" are in the ingredients list, it contains trans fat and is not a good choice. If you can read all of the ingredients in the product, and they each sound like real food, it's probably a decent choice. If you want to know more about the product, look at the nutrition-facts label for total calories, grams of fat, sugars, and sodium. Just keep in mind that real food is pretty easy to spot, and you won't have to try very hard or do much detective work to find it. If you find yourself analyzing a food and trying to decide if it's healthy or not, it probably isn't.

Keeping Food Fresh

Processed foods are filled with additives and preservatives like nitrates and salt to keep them fresh for months and even years. When you eat real food, the chemical soup of preservatives isn't present to keep the food fresh. Remember, real food rots. When there are tons of vitamins, minerals, and enzymes still present in food, bacteria and other microorganisms are naturally attracted to your food to break it down.

As a result, some creative strategies are required to make sure that you eat the food before it spoils, or store it in a way that keeps it fresh so your hard-earned food dollars don't get tossed in the trash or the compost heap.

As we've discussed, meal planning each week and shopping for only the fresh fruits and vegetables that you plan to use right away in your meal plan is the simplest and most effective strategy for preventing food waste and for keeping food fresh, because you've created a specific plan to use the food up before it spoils.

You can store foods on the counter, in your pantry or cupboards, in the fridge, or in the freezer to keep them fresh. The best place to store food depends largely on how soon you're planning to use it up. Food storage also depends on what type of food it is and how it's been prepared before you buy it.

Fruits and vegetables are highly perishable in their fresh and natural state, so learning how to keep them fresh will ensure that you get the most out of them. One thing to keep in mind is that fresh fruits and vegetables are most nutritious and flavorful when picked ripe and eaten as soon as possible after they are picked.

Store most fresh fruits and vegetables in the produce-crisper drawers in your refrigerator at 38 to 40 degrees Fahrenheit. If you have two crisper drawers in your fridge, keep fresh fruits in one and fresh vegetables in the other. If you have the option, set the humidity of your fruit and vegetable drawers to high humidity, or 80 to 100 percent relative humidity. Because they are filled with water, setting the humidity to low and allowing the dry fridge air into your crisper drawers will actually dry out your fresh produce and cause it to spoil faster. Think about the sprinklers in the produce cases in the grocery store for leafy greens and other vegetables—these keep the veggies moist and fresh.

Many fruits like apples, pears, and melon produce ethylene gas, which causes fruits and vegetables to ripen faster and over-ripen in the fridge. This is why it's helpful to separate fruits from vegetables and leafy greens in your refrigerator produce-crisper drawers. To help preserve delicate veggies like leafy greens, salad greens, and herbs, you can purchase special produce bags that protect them, hold in moisture, and keep them fresher longer. If you have room in your fridge, you can also store bunches of fresh herbs like parsley and cilantro in a cup of water to keep them fresh and moist.

To keep produce fresher longer, don't wash produce before you store it—just pick it or buy it and store it in its natural state. The one exception is berries. To keep fresh raspberries, blackberries, blueberries, and strawberries fresh, a client of mine shared a great tip. When you get them home, put the berries in a bowl filled with one part white vinegar and ten parts water to kill mold spores and bacteria. Then drain off all the water and store the berries in a bowl in the fridge until you eat them up.

Many fruits and vegetables are best stored in the fridge, but some are not. Peaches, plums, and apricots are best stored in a paper bag at room temperature until they are ripe and ready to eat. Fresh tomatoes and melons can also be stored on your counter. Once they are ripe, eat them, cut them up and freeze them, or put them in the fruit drawer in the fridge. Bananas can be stored on the counter as well, until ripe. When they are ripe, cut them up and store them in a freezer bag in the freezer to use later in pancake or bread recipes or smoothies. Winter squash, pumpkins, sweet potatoes, white potatoes, onions, and garlic can all be stored at room temperature in a cool, dry place, like in your pantry, to keep them fresh.

As a general rule, most fresh fruits and vegetables last about a week if stored properly. Some produce won't last a full week, and some will keep fresh for longer, but having a plan to use up fresh food within a week of buying it is a good plan to ensure that your food stays fresh, vibrant, and full of nutrition. If produce is ripe and you can't use it all right away, often the best option is to freeze it. Wash and cut fruit and berries, then put them in a freezer bag in the freezer to keep them fresh until you're ready to use them. If fruits are prone to stick together, like strawberries, blueberries, and others, then freeze them on a baking sheet and transfer them to a freezer bag once they are frozen. Most fresh vegetables can be frozen quite easily as well. Simply wash and cut them as you would for a recipe, blanch them briefly in boiling water to prevent freezer burn, then put them in a freezer bag and freeze until you're ready to use them. When freezing fruits or vegetables, just be sure to write the contents and date on the bag so you can keep track of how long they've been in your freezer. Frozen fruits and vegetables should remain fresh for six months to a year in the freezer.

Other perishables like meat, poultry, fish, eggs, milk, cheeses, yogurt, and many condiments also need to be refrigerated or frozen to keep them fresh. For dairy products and eggs, store them in the fridge and keep an eye on the "sell-by date," and use them up before that date, if possible. If you buy meat, poultry, or fish frozen, keep them frozen until you're ready to use them, and unthaw them overnight in the refrigerator. You can also buy meat, poultry, or fish fresh. If you do this, cook them up within a couple days or put them in the freezer right away. To prevent freezer burn, one trick is to wrap them in freezer paper, then put them in a freezer bag. If you happen to own one, using freezer bags specially designed for a vacuum sealer is even better at sealing foods for the freezer and preventing freezer burn. Just remember to label the contents and date so you know how long they have been in the freezer. Meat, poultry, and fish should last about six to twelve months in the freezer.

While produce and perishables need to be carefully stored to keep them fresh, other real foods like whole grains, beans and legumes, nuts and seeds, oils, as well as herbs and spices also need to be stored properly to ensure that they remain fresh and nutritious.

Since whole grains have the whole grain intact, including the bran and the germ, which contain oils, they don't last as long as refined or processed grains. It's best to buy whole grains from bulk bins or in one- to two-pound packages so that they are fresh when you buy them. To prevent whole grains from going rancid, store them in a cool, dry place like your pantry cupboard in air-tight containers like glass jars, and use them up often. Ground grains or whole-grain flours should be stored in airtight jars and kept in your fridge or freezer, if you have room, to keep them fresh and prevent bugs from getting into them. Whole grains and whole-grain flours should last three to six months if stored properly. Cooked whole grains and baked goods made from whole-grain flours can be stored in airtight containers in your fridge for up to five days and frozen for about six months.

Dried beans, lentils, and split peas should be stored in airtight containers, like glass jars, in a cool, dry place. Replace them every three to six months, as fresh beans cook faster, are softer when cooked, and are easier to digest. If you make extra beans, you can store them in the fridge for three to four days to use in other recipes, or you can freeze leftover beans in freezer-safe bags or containers for up to six months for later use.

Dried herbs and spices should also be stored in airtight containers in a cool, dry place. When you purchase them in their containers or in bulk, be sure to mark the date of purchase so you know how long they've been in your cupboard. Dried herbs and spices lose their flavor and pizzazz long before most people toss them and replace them with new ones. Dried herbs and ground spices should be replaced every six to twelve months to ensure that they are fresh and doing their job in the kitchen.

Learning to store real food in a way that keeps it fresh is essential to having fresh ingredients for healthy and delicious meals and snacks.

Meal Preparation and Cooking

Now that you've got a meal plan and a strategy for shopping for the food you need, meal preparation and cooking is much simpler and a lot more fun. When your pantry, cupboards, fridge, and freezer are stocked with real food, you can be creative and enjoy the process of preparing healthy meals.

Chefs use the term *mise en place*, which literally translates to "everything in its place." This way of preparing meals and cooking is extremely helpful because it encourages you to cut and prepare all of your ingredients first, then start cooking. When you're starting to prepare more meals at home, try new recipes, and increase your cooking repertoire of skills and dishes, cutting fresh fruits and vegetables first for your dishes and having all of your ingredients out and ready to go will make a big difference. It's a systematic way of cooking that saves you time, frustration, and allows you to focus on the task at hand when you're cooking.

To make meal preparation and cooking more efficient, tasty, and nutritious, it's helpful to learn some basic cutting, food-preparation, and cooking techniques.

Cutting techniques

▶ **Chiffonade**: This technique is perfect for making long, thin strips of leafy greens or herbs. Stack the leafy greens on top of each other and then roll tightly lengthwise. Hold the rolled leafy greens tightly and slice across every eighth inch to quarter inch.

▶ **Chopping:** This technique is great when no particular size or shape is needed, like for stir-fry dishes. Use a chef's knife to cut the food into appropriate-sized pieces for your dish.

▶ **Dicing:** This technique is more precise than chopping. When you dice food, slice the food into long, thin strips, then cut across to make eighth-inch to quarter-inch cubes. Dicing is often used to cut onions, peppers, and other vegetables.

▶ **Julienne:** Also known as matchsticks, julienne-cut vegetables are used for sushi, spring rolls, and other dishes where matchstick-sized vegetables are needed. To create julienne-cut vegetables like carrots or cucumber, simply make eighth-inch-thick slices diagonally down the vegetable. Then cut each slice into eighth-inch-square matchstick pieces.

▶ **Mincing:** This is a great cutting technique to use for strongly flavored foods like garlic, ginger, and hot peppers. To mince foods, use a chef's knife to cut them into flat pieces, then rock the knife back and forth to create finely cut pieces.

▶ **Shredding:** Use a box grater or food processor to shred foods like vegetables or cheeses into thin strips. Shredded vegetables are great on salads or in baked goods, and you can vary the shred size by using a different blade on the box grater or food processor.

▶ **Slicing:** This technique is pretty general and simply means cutting food into strips, wedges, rings, rounds, or slices. The type of slicing required for different foods is often called out in the recipe. Making appropriate slices for different foods adds character, flavor, visual appeal, and texture to dishes. Apples, for example, can be cut into thin slices, wedges, or rings.

▶ **Zesting:** This technique uses a zester or microplane grater to grate the outer peel of citrus fruit to make orange or lemon zest. The same technique can also be used to grate whole nutmeg and ginger root finely for use in various dishes.

Food-preparation techniques

▶ **Freezing:** Buying extra produce when it's in season or making intentional leftovers and freezing them is a great way to preserve food. Most foods containing liquid, like soups, stews, dips, pesto, and applesauce, freeze well and are good up to six months in the freezer. You can also blanch and freeze fresh vegetables or fresh berries on cookie sheets and transfer them into a freezer container or bag once frozen.

▶ **Marinating:** This technique is perfect for tenderizing and flavoring meat and some vegetable dishes. Use an acidic liquid like lemon juice or vinegar or a salty base like tamari. Pour the liquid over the meat or vegetable dish and allow the flavors to combine. Store covered in the refrigerator until ready to use.

▶ **Pureeing:** When puréed or blended, cooked soups, steamed vegetables, or frozen fruit and other smoothie ingredients turn into smooth and creamy liquids. Use a blender or immersion blender for puréeing foods.

▶ **Rinsing:** Some foods like lentils and quinoa need to be rinsed prior to cooking to remove dust and the plant's natural bitter outer coating. Use a fine wire mesh strainer and rinse these foods until the water runs clear.

▶ **Soaking:** This technique is great for rehydrating and softening foods like beans, whole grains, nuts, seeds, dried fruit, and sun-dried tomatoes. Put whatever food you'd like to soak into a bowl and cover with purified water. Leave the bowl on your counter at room temperature for anywhere from twenty minutes for sun-dried tomatoes to overnight for brown rice or dried beans.

Cooking techniques

▶ **Baking:** This technique is perfect for meats, fish, hearty vegetables, and baked goods like breads, cookies, muffins, and many more. Heat the oven to the required temperature and bake on a baking sheet or in a baking dish until cooked through.

▶ **Boiling:** If you want to reheat food, cook pasta, or quickly cook greens or other vegetables on the stove, add water or stock to a saucepan. Set the stove to medium to medium-high heat, and allow the liquid to boil. Next, add the food and cook until done.

▶ **Braising:** This technique is great for tough cuts of meat and some hearty vegetables like parsnips. Sauté the food until it's cooked through, then add a flavorful liquid, cover, and simmer until the food absorbs the liquid.

▶ **Broiling:** This is great for some fish and cuts of meat. Move an oven rack to the top shelf and turn the oven on to "broil." Place the food in a baking dish on the top oven rack to broil.

▶ **Dehydrating:** Foods are sometimes "cooked" at low temperatures to dry them out. This preserves a lot of the nutrition like vitamins and enzymes in the food that is lost when cooked at high temperatures. Apples, pineapple, cherries, apricots, carrots, sweet potatoes, and other fruits, vegetables, and even meats can be dehydrated on dehydrator sheets to preserve them.

▶ **Double boiling:** This technique is very similar to boiling, except when you double boil foods, the water in the saucepan doesn't come into contact with the food. Use a double boiler pan or metal mixing bowl and place it on top of the boiling water. Add food to reheat, chocolate, or whatever you want to gently heat and cook until heated through.

▶ **Dry roasting:** Place food like pumpkin seeds or coated almonds in a single layer on a baking sheet in the oven to roast. Shake the baking sheet during roasting to prevent burning. You can also dry roast nuts or seeds in a skillet on the stove. Jostle the food frequently to prevent burning and remove when nuts or seeds are slightly browned.

▶ **Grilling:** This technique is perfect on a hot summer day when you don't want to turn on the stove or oven inside. Meat, fish, shrimp, and vegetables are great when cooked on the grill. Place small pieces of meat, poultry, seafood, or cut vegetables in a grill basket or on skewers to prevent them from falling through.

▶ **Sautéing:** You can sauté foods in a heated skillet with oil, water, or some other liquid like broth or white wine. Sautéing is great for vegetables and greens and is a quick and easy cooking technique. Keep foods in the skillet moving to prevent sticking or burning, and make sure that all ingredients are prepared and ready to add.

▶ **Steaming:** This technique is great for cooking vegetables to crisp-tender when pierced with a fork. Vegetables tend to maintain more nutritional value when steamed versus many other cooking methods. Add some water to the bottom of a saucepan, add a metal steaming basket, and then add the vegetables. Put a lid on the pan to retain moisture, and set a timer.

When it's time to prepare a meal, look at your meal plan to see what you've planned to make. Get out your meal-planning binder or cookbook if you need to look up recipes and directions. Next, get out the needed ingredients for your meal and get to work preparing the meal. Start with the dish that will take the longest, and move on to the next one when that one is cooking. Coordinating the timing of dishes to produce a meal that is done at the same time takes some practice. Stick with it, and you'll figure out a rhythm that works for you.

When you're cooking beans or grains like rice or quinoa, set a timer. Just set the timer and work on all the other food preparation until the beans or grains are cooked. To download the Bean Cooking Guide and the Whole Grain Cooking Guide, go to www.erinharner.com/real-food-resources/. This frees you up to work on other dishes or set the table. You can also use a kitchen timer to time how long it takes you to do certain things like chopping, sautéing, baking, and such, so you get an idea of how long things take. This ensures everything is done at about the same time.

Once you've prepared your meal, you have two choices on how to serve it. You can serve it family-style, where you bring all of the dishes to the table and serve yourself. This works well and allows everyone at the meal to take the amount of food that they would like to eat. The downside of serving meals this way is that you can go back for more as many times as you want. Since your meal is full of healthy real food, the quantity that you eat matters less, but having more food right in front of you can trick your brain and your stomach into thinking that you're still hungry when you've had enough.

The other option for serving food that works quite well is to serve it from the kitchen. Each person can take their plate to the kitchen and serve themselves, or one person can serve all of the plates and deliver them to the table. Either way, second helpings are a walk away instead of right in front of you, so it forces you to check in with your body to see if you're still hungry before you get up. The key with this strategy is to serve enough food the first time and enjoy what you have on your plate.

After you've eaten, you may have some leftovers. Store your leftovers in airtight containers in the fridge for up to three or four days. If you don't anticipate eating them before they spoil in the fridge, you can put leftovers in freezer-safe containers or bags and store them in the freezer for three to six months and simply take them out, thaw them, heat them, and eat them whenever you need a quick ready-made meal.

CHAPTER 9

Real Food When You're Not at Home

"When walking, walk. When eating, eat." –Zen Proverb

There are two main places you eat: at home and somewhere else. At home, you typically make meals in your kitchen and eat in the kitchen or dining room. The purpose of this book is to show you how to make eating real food simple and doable for your lifestyle, no matter where you are. Remember that real food is exactly the same whether you're at home or not.

Situations where you eat away from home include when you're on the go, like in the car, at a party, picnic, potluck, at a meeting, traveling for work, on vacation, or out at a restaurant. Eating healthy real food when you're not at home can be a challenge because you lose some control over how the food is prepared, unless you make it and bring it with you. Studies have shown that average Americans eat more than 50 percent of their meals away from home. The problem with this is that we spend more money, consume more fat, sugar, and salt, and eat more food when other people prepare our meals for us.

Hopefully the previous chapters have inspired you to cook at home more and eat out less. But no matter where you are, just remember the principles of a healthy real-food diet and let them guide you to make smart choices. Having a solid understanding of what real food is and what real food is not will help you navigate the incredibly confusing food environment when you're not at home.

Client Story:

Peggy is an environmental analyst, wife, and mother of two active teenage boys. Before going through the Get Real in 8 Weeks Program, Peggy was "flying by the seat of [her] pants and not making good choices for meals." She made some big changes to her diet with my help previously when she was diagnosed with Celiac disease and eliminated gluten from her diet but found that she was slipping back into eating out three to four times per week and eating a lot of sugary snacks.

Throughout our time working together, Peggy implemented the tools that she learned and after just eight short weeks, she is now feeling "a lot more confident and less guilty" because she is eating more real food at home. Also, when she goes out to eat, she is making better choices and relying on real food for snacks instead of processed foods. She now has "more energy, less stress, less pain, less inflammation, and feels a lot better in [her] body!"

Real Food on the Go

The best strategy for healthy eating on the go is to bring real food with you. You should have a good idea about your schedule ahead of time, so be sure this is included in your weekly meal plan. This will ensure that you have what you need when you need it, and also that you don't fuel your body the same place you fuel your car or wind up pulling through a fast-food restaurant drive-through.

Whenever you leave home, whether you're headed to work, an appointment, to exercise, to a party, or whatever—always take a water bottle with you. That way you have access to water all the time to keep you well hydrated and ward off cravings. Also, take meals or snacks with you that are quick and easy to pack, sturdy, and don't need to be chilled unless you have a container to keep them cold, an ice pack, or a fridge at your destination. You could pack leftovers for lunch or a snack. Or you can make something up quickly to take with you, like cut vegetables, trail mix, or a sandwich. Produce or whole-grain foods paired with lean proteins or healthy fats make great snacks and mini-meals.

Remember, the easiest and most budget-friendly way to eat a real-food diet on the go is to bring it with you. To make it even easier, you can prepack snacks in appropriate portions in small bags or containers when you bring the food home from the store. That way, they will be ready to grab and go when you're running out the door. In your cooler or bag, pack any of the following real-food snacks in appropriate amounts based on how long you will be gone:

- Apple or pear slices with nut butter
- Applesauce with almonds
- Banana with nut butter
- Brown-rice cakes with nut butter
- Carrot sticks, celery, or cucumber with yogurt dip or hummus
- Fruit and nut granola
- Hard-boiled egg with fresh-cut vegetables

▶ Homemade granola bar or energy bar

▶ Orange, plum, or peach with a small handful of almonds or walnuts

▶ Premade fruit smoothie

▶ Real-food bar made with dried fruit, nuts, and/or seeds

▶ Sandwich (nut butter and no-sugar-added jam or other)

▶ Soaked almonds with cinnamon

▶ Trail mix made with raw nuts, seeds, and dried fruit

▶ Whole-grain or flaxseed crackers with hummus, nut butter, or canned salmon

▶ Yogurt with berries and nuts

If you do a lot of driving, you can even keep some of these nonperishable snacks in your car so they are always there when you need them. If it's really hot, though, it's better to just bring snacks with you, since foods like nuts and seeds will go rancid. If you work a desk job, you can keep some healthy real food in your office for when you need a snack; that way you won't have to remember to bring it every day. Whole-grain crackers, brown-rice cakes, nut butters, applesauce cups, trail mix, and whole fresh fruit like apples and pears keep pretty well at room temperature and will help you avoid a mid-afternoon run to the vending machine, cafeteria, or coffee shop.

If you're attending an event like a party, picnic, dish-to-pass, or potluck, the best solution to ensure that you're going to be able to find healthy real food is to bring it yourself. Don't rely on the host or other attendees to make real food, because there is a good chance that they won't. In this case, bring a veggie tray with hummus, fresh-fruit skewers, whole-grain salad, bean salad, or a sweet potato salad (see recipes in appendix C). That way, you will have something healthy to eat, and other people attending the event will be appreciative that there is something healthy to eat as well. Whenever you're on the go, the best option is to take advantage of what is in your well-stocked real-food kitchen first, and bring that with you.

Real Food When You're Eating Out

Sometimes packing food to bring with you simply isn't possible. In these cases, your food options are dependent on what's immediately available to you or made by others. You may need to rely on restaurants, cafeterias, or grocery stores to provide food for you. In this case, there are some additional things to consider. When you're eating out, there seems to be unlimited options, but your ability to put together real-food meals relies on you choosing a place that serves real food.

If you're short on time and looking for a fast and healthy real-food meal, you can easily turn the grocery store into your real-food fast-food stop. This works because grocery stores stock real food. There are lots of great real-food options at the grocery store, and there is a lot of junk, so know what you are going into the store for before you walk through the door. Start in the produce section. Vegetables such as carrots, cherry tomatoes, sugar snap peas, as well as precut veggies like bell peppers, celery, or cucumbers are great to buy to dip into something protein-rich like black bean dip, hummus, nut butter, or even guacamole to make the base of a snack or meal. Fruits such as apples, bananas, grapes, oranges, peaches, plums, nectarines, and berries are quick to grab and easy to take with you. In the bulk section, you can usually find a good selection of raw nuts and seeds and dried fruit. If you tolerate dairy, you can also grab unsweetened yogurt, cottage cheese, or cheese to round out your meal.

Grocery stores that have prepared-foods sections can also be really handy if you're in a hurry to find real food on the go. Often, you can find quinoa salad, pasta salad, vegetable sushi, or roasted chickens. It takes some creativity to come up with a quick and delicious meal from the grocery store, but you can be sure that it's real food because you assembled it yourself. An added bonus of this strategy is that it often costs less to put a meal together yourself from the grocery store than it would cost to buy it at a restaurant. Assembling real-food meals at a grocery store is somewhere in between making it at home and taking it with you, and eating out.

If you decide to eat out at a restaurant, diner, cafeteria, or some other place that serves food, it's really helpful to make a few decisions before you even pull into the parking lot. Remember the 90-10 Rule? Is this meal part of the healthy 90 percent or the 10 percent splurge? Before you even make a decision about where you're going to go, be very clear about your intention for the meal. If you decide that it's part of the 10 percent, order whatever you are hungry for and simply enjoy it. If your meal is part of the healthy real-food 90 percent, then you have some more choices to make.

The biggest thing to remember when eating out is that restaurants and places that serve food have profits at the top of their priority list, not your health. Because of this, restaurants have really good marketing teams to get you to buy the most profitable items. They have a lot of options on their menus, which can overwhelm you if you're looking for something healthy. And the menu may even trick you into thinking that you want something that you really don't.

Another challenge with most restaurants is that they use a lot more salt, sugar, fats, and oils than you would ever use at home if you were preparing the food yourself. They also use chemicals like MSG to give food a savory flavor. MSG has been shown to have negative effects in study after study, but restaurants keep using it. Would you keep MSG in your cupboard at home? I don't think so.

Another problem with food served at most restaurants or other establishments is portion size. If you were to serve yourself a filling portion of pasta at home, it would likely be a fraction of the amount of pasta served to you at a restaurant. Because restaurants typically serve much larger portions of food than you would ever serve yourself at home, it's really important to be conscious of your body and when you're full. Just remember that proper portion sizes are exactly the same when you're eating out as they are at home—use your hand as a guide. One serving of whole grains, pasta, or fruit is about the size of your closed fist; one serving of meat, poultry, or fish is about the size of your open palm; and one serving of nuts, seeds, nut butters, fats, or oils should be no larger than your thumb.

When you combine the high-salt, high-fat, high-sugar, calorie-dense food served at most restaurants with gigantic portion sizes, it's not a stretch to see how eating out frequently can lead to weight gain and other health challenges quite quickly; unless, of course, you're diligent about consciously making healthy choices.

The next decision to make is where you'll go out to eat. It's pretty simple to find real food at most restaurants if you look for it, or if you deliberately choose a place that serves healthy food. Ethnic restaurants tend to have much more real food on their menus than fast-food restaurants, diners, or burger joints.

After you've made the decision about where you're going out to eat, check in with your body to figure out what you're hungry for before you even open the menu. Then open the menu and see if they have anything similar to what you want. It's easy to get carried away by high-fat, high-carb, and high-sugar restaurant meals, so try to listen to what your body wants, and order that. To help you make better choices when eating out, take a look at the following ethnic cuisines for some healthier options at each:

- **American:** Try choosing steamed, broiled, boiled, or grilled dishes; or tomato-based dishes like salads, chicken, or vegetables instead of fried, breaded, creamy, buttery, or cheesy dishes like macaroni and cheese, French fries, breaded and fried chicken, or burgers.

- **Chinese:** Try choosing stir-fried veggies or steamed veggies, lean meat or tofu, and brown rice, if they have it. You could also try a noodle dish with veggies and meat or tofu. Try to stay away from sweet-and-sour dishes, tempura, and deep-fried dishes like egg rolls.

- **Japanese:** Try sushi, sashimi, miso soup, teriyaki dishes, steamed veggies, and brown rice or udon noodles. Stay away from tempura dishes and sushi or sashimi with creamy fillings like cream cheese.

- **Indian:** Give tandoori dishes, lentil dahl, chana masala, veggie curries, or brown basmati rice a try. Avoid rich meat curries, dishes with a heavy cream base, and fried foods like samosas and pakora.

- **Greek:** Try choosing Greek salad, dolmades, hummus, meat souvlaki, fish dishes, fruit, and Greek yogurt. Stay away from foods like fried falafel, meatballs, sausages, and baklava.

▶ **Italian:** Choose pasta with tomato-based sauces, risotto, gnocci, veggie pizza, grilled chicken or fish, or salad. Try to avoid pasta with creamy or butter-based sauces, lasagna, pizza with sausage or pepperoni, and high-fat desserts.

▶ **Mexican:** Try choosing burritos or fajitas with black beans, chicken, and vegetables, corn tortillas, guacamole, salsa, brown rice, if they have it, or veggie chili. Stay away from tortilla chips, fried shells, sour cream, non-vegetarian refried beans, meat chili, and chimichangas.

There are a number of other strategies you can use to make eating out healthier. Try making savvy substitutions of vegetables or a side salad for fries, chips, or potatoes, brown rice for white rice, or fresh-cut vegetables instead of a breadbasket. Another strategy is to design your own meal from what is on the menu. This is especially effective if you have special dietary needs like gluten-free, dairy-free, or vegetarian and the restaurant doesn't specifically cater to what you're looking for. Simply figure out what you want, take a look at the menu, and find some items on the menu that you'd like for your meal. Ask politely when you order, and the restaurant will likely be willing to make you a customized meal to fit your needs.

To control portion size so you're not tempted to eat four servings of pasta in one sitting, for example, try splitting an entrée, ordering an appetizer and side salad for your dinner, or get half of your serving wrapped to go before the wait staff serves you, so you're not even tempted to eat the whole thing. Just remember that it is possible to eat healthy real food when you're on the go if you plan ahead and make conscious choices.

CHAPTER 10

Simplify and Streamline Healthy Eating

"And in the end it's not the years in your life that count. It's the life in your years." –Abraham Lincoln

It takes twenty-one days to create a habit. What you have to think about at first becomes routine in three short weeks. It's like brushing your teeth. When you implement what you've learned in this book and harness the power of the daily routine, you will cultivate healthy habits that support your health, boost your energy, and ensure that you and your family eat real food and are well cared for.

Keep it simple. Incorporate the simple strategies and information in this book and you'll have a plan that works every time. You will avoid mealtime overwhelm by having groceries in the fridge, an organized kitchen with the tools and appliances you need, a weekly meal plan, and the skills, knowledge, and confidence needed to prepare healthy meals quickly. This peace of mind goes far beyond mealtime—it will result in you being calmer and will unlock a lot of time and energy to do other things you love.

Healthy meals do not have to be complicated or take a long time to prepare. They can be simple, delicious, and meet your needs perfectly. Preparing real-food meals in under twenty or thirty minutes every day of the week starts with a plan and has a lot to do with tips and tricks to simplify and streamline the process.

To save time in the kitchen, one of the simplest and easiest things to do is to make a big dinner each night and pack leftovers to take for lunch the next day. This allows you to make one meal and get two out of it. Not to mention, lunch is generally the least healthy meal of the day for most, so by taking a good dinner for lunch, it ensures that you have a healthy lunch each day, instead of just grabbing whatever is available. Packing lunch as you're putting away the dinner dishes also saves time in the morning—all you have to do is grab your lunch and go.

Cooking once and eating multiple meals from the same dish, like beans or grains, can also make cooking faster and easier. For example, soak and cook brown rice one night for dinner. Eat some leftover brown rice with the dish you're taking for lunch the next day. For dinner, try making rice and beans, stuffed peppers, or vegetable fried rice from the rice you already cooked. This will cut down on meal prep time significantly, since brown rice takes about an hour to cook the first time and only a few minutes to heat up with a new dish. When you soak and cook extra beans or whole grains, they can also be frozen in freezer-safe containers or bags to use when you need them in the same way for different dishes.

You can also make extra-large quantities of dinner entrées and freeze some of the leftovers for those nights when you're really busy and pressed for time. Raw meat patties, casseroles, lasagna, soups, and stews all freeze well.

Plan to eat the frozen entrées you made previously in your meal plan for the week. Since you should know ahead of time which nights will be really busy, you can pull them out of the freezer in the morning and defrost them in the fridge during the day. When you get home, your dinner is already defrosted, and all you have to do is heat it up, and it's ready to eat. When you make a dinner that would freeze well, just be sure to make extra to make this work. This is an especially effective strategy if you're cooking for one or two people; that way you're not eating the same leftovers day after day.

If you are really pressed for time or know ahead that you're going to be really busy, you can also plan a fresh meal like pasta with a tomato-based sauce, a sandwich on hearty bread, or tortillas with beans, rice, lettuce, and tomatoes. These can all be prepared in less than ten minutes and are fairly healthy options.

Another great option when time in the evening is short is to use a slow cooker. Slow cookers are great because they allow you to cook a full meal when you're not even home. Soups, stews, chili, and roasts can all be cooked successfully in a slow cooker. Just be sure that your slow cooker has variable temperature settings, including "warm," and a cook timer. You could even make slow-cooked oatmeal and cook it overnight, so it's hot and ready for breakfast in the morning.

Add some zing to spice up meals using spices and herbs. You can prepare the exact same dish using different herbs and spices, and it will taste entirely different. For example, you could cook and season a sliced chicken breast with curry powder to give it an Indian flavor, cook the chicken in the same way with Italian herbs and serve it with pasta, or cook it exactly the same way with a Mexican spice blend to use in tacos or tortillas. You can also use condiments to give the same foods different flavors. Just remember, when it comes to condiments, herbs, spices, and salt—less really is more. Just lightly flavor your food so you can taste the goodness, don't overpower it.

Another technique that makes preparing healthy meals quick and easy is to precut vegetables ahead of time. If you've planned out that you need a bunch of carrots cut for the week, you can precut them however you need them and store them in the fridge. You could also precut vegetables and make mixes for different dishes and freeze them as well. An example is for stir-fries. You could cut some bell peppers, onions, carrots, broccoli and whatever else you like to put in your stir-fry, mix all the veggies together, and store in the freezer in a freezer-safe bag or container until you're ready to use them.

Precut veggies also make great snacks during the week. You can cut up carrots, celery, bell peppers, and whatever other vegetables you like to eat raw and keep them in the fridge to snack on. If they are precut and ready to eat, you are far more likely to reach for vegetables instead of chips or something else. They are also convenient to throw in with your (or your kids') lunch. You can do the same thing with salads, too. Prepare a big bag of salad ahead of time and store it in produce bags to keep it fresh. It takes the same amount of time to make ten salads as it does one, so do it all at once and save yourself a ton of time and make it convenient to eat all week.

You can also juice vegetables and use the pulp for other dishes like lentil burgers and black bean burgers. Juicing fresh vegetables is incredibly healthy and a great way to get extremely nutrient-dense vegetables in a glass. When you juice, however, the fibrous pulp from the vegetables is usually discarded. Instead of just tossing or composting the pulp, get creative and use it for other dishes. When vegetables like leafy greens, cucumbers, carrots, or celery are no longer great for eating fresh, just turn them into juice.

Smoothies are another quick and easy grab-and-go snack or mini-meal. They can be made healthy, protein-rich, and nutrient-dense, which is a great combination for breakfast. Add some frozen or fresh fruit; unsweetened Greek yogurt, pure protein powder like whey, quinoa, or pea protein powder, or a green or superfood blend; and some liquid, like unsweetened almond milk, water, or a splash of fruit juice for a delicious drink to go. If you're up to it, add some kale, spinach, or other leafy green to give your smoothie some added healthy punch. If you use blueberries or blackberries in the smoothie, you won't even notice the greens. Smoothies can be premade and taken with you for later as well. Don't be afraid to get creative and experiment.

If you prepare meals for people with different dietary needs, like gluten-free, dairy-free, low-glycemic, Paleolithic, vegan, or whatever—cooking meals can get tricky. The best thing to do is to get everyone on the same page so you don't end up making different dishes for different preferences and needs each day. This can get really frustrating and creates a lot of extra work and extra dishes. Instead of making different dishes or meals for different needs or picky eaters, compromise by making the same base meal or by emphasizing real foods that work with different needs and preferences. For example, if you're serving gluten-free, vegetarians, and meat-eating people the same meal, you could make gluten-free pasta made from brown rice for everyone, a side of vegetables, and pasta sauce that works for all three preferences. Then you could make gluten-free ground turkey meatballs for the meat eaters and black bean "meatballs" for the vegetarians. This will require some creativity at first; just be sure that you plan meals ahead, and it will become a lot easier.

Hydration is also crucial, and the simplest way to stay hydrated is to carry a water bottle with you at all times. Quit wasting money and precious resources on bottled water, and start bringing your own. Add essential oils like lemon, orange, peppermint, or lavender, a squirt of lemon juice, or a slice of cucumber to your water to make it more appealing, if needed. Just remember to take your water bottle with you wherever you go and do what you can to stay hydrated. Mix it up and keep it interesting.

Despite your best intentions and having a weekly meal plan, sometimes you're going to need to make healthy upgrades to foods as you go or swap ingredients out on the fly if you don't have them. Don't worry about it, just replace ingredients with what you have that's healthy. For example, if your recipe calls for arugula and you couldn't find it, depending on the dish, you could just leave it out, replace it with an herb like cilantro, or replace it with another green like spinach. It's not important that your meals are perfect or you follow every recipe to the tee; all that matters is that you get tasty, healthy meals on the table.

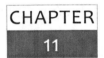

Your Personalized Plan for More Energy, Less Stress, and Healthy Meals in Minutes

"Happiness is when what you think, what you say, and what you do are in harmony." –Mahatma Gandhi

Throughout this book, you learned a number of mind-set strategies to set you up for a healthy diet and lifestyle. You learned what real food is and what it's not. You learned how to plan meals, shop for real food at various places, prepare healthy real-food meals in your kitchen, and even tips and strategies for making healthy eating even simpler. In addition, you learned that making healthy choices at home and on the go every day of the week depends on having a plan to make it work.

True energy, nourishment, and fulfillment don't happen by accident. They are a direct result of creating and intentionally following a well-laid plan to feed and nourish your body with real food. When you combine fresh, healthy real food and the real-food staples in your pantry with your loving preparation and cooking skills, magic happens.

The two key elements of a plan are *what* and *when*. Since your plan is dependent on time and you only have so much of it, using an electronic or paper calendar will make your life a whole lot easier. It may take some getting used to, but if you're busy and you want to fit something in and remember to do it, it has to be on your calendar or things will come up, and it will get pushed aside. Every Sunday night, I put together our weekly meal plan, schedule for the week, and my priorities for the week. Then my husband and I sit down and go through the week together so we know what to expect and what's coming. This weekly planning meeting with everyone in the house (even if it's just you) to discuss the weekly schedule, meal plan, and what you're doing for fun that week is one of the most powerful habits I've ever created. It is also a great opportunity to get feedback or input on your meal plan from your family. Start planning ahead and directing each week and day instead of reacting to it as it comes. This one strategy alone will help you radically free up energy and reduce your stress.

Throughout this book, you started to create your personalized plan for more energy, less stress, and healthy meals in minutes. Let's review the elements of your plan to tie together what you've learned:

1. Decide to get healthy by eating wholesome real-food meals.
2. Get support to get you started and keep you motivated and on track.
3. Clean out your kitchen and stock it with real food and essential kitchen tools.
4. Make a list of healthy real-food meals that you and your family enjoy.
5. Create a weekly meal plan each week and write what you need on your grocery list.
6. Go food shopping each week after you create your meal plan and stick to your list.

7. Hold a planning meeting each week to discuss and prepare for the week ahead.

8. Follow your meal plan throughout the week to get healthy meals on the table in minutes.

9. Enjoy having more energy, less stress, and renewed confidence.

10. Repeat steps 5 through 9 each week.

When you live authentically and you put time and energy into what really matters to you, it's a recipe for a happy, fulfilled life. Instead of constantly trying to find balance in your life, find focus instead. When you do something, do it. When you eat, eat (and chew). When you make dinner, make dinner. We have gotten to be master multitaskers, but when you quit multitasking and start single-tasking and focus on one thing at a time, you'll do what you're doing faster and better. Doing one thing at a time and being present will also increase your enjoyment of the activity, whether it's shopping, cooking, or eating dinner.

The other great benefit of planning and focusing is that your ability to set boundaries increases. When you know what is important to you, it makes it much easier to say "yes" to the right things and "not right now" to the other things that don't really matter. By being intentional and conserving your energy for the stuff that's important to you, it sparks confidence and an incredible feeling of control in your life. Creating alignment between what's important to you and what you actually do makes you feel good.

We are creatures of habit. Throughout this book, I showed you how to cultivate healthy habits, eat a wholesome real-food diet, and make healthy choices no matter where you are. These new healthy habits create a positive feedback loop in your life—

eating healthy makes you feel good which makes you want to continue eating real food. Feeling good and full of energy creates a ripple effect throughout your life, as it will encourage you to do other healthy things like exercise and movement, rest, and more self-care.

Diet and exercise go hand-in-hand. To achieve optimal health and feel great, you need both. Exercise and movement make you feel strong, flexible, and confident. Find exercise that you love to do, and do more of that. Getting your body in shape makes you want to eat more healthy food and creates a positive cycle of feeling good for the long haul, which will help to keep you on track. Also, when your body and mind are fed with real-food fuel, your basic need for sustenance is met, and you are much more equipped to open up to other avenues of nourishment in your life to create true happiness, contentment, and fulfillment. After all, all the healthy food in the world will never be able to fill a void in your life in the areas of movement, rest and relaxation, connection, or self-care.

Having consistent downtime is also essential to having more energy and less stress. It allows your body and mind a chance to rejuvenate and recover from the demands of your busy life. Plan for time each week when you can relax and unwind. This time is for you, and just knowing that it's in your schedule, will keep you grounded.

One activity that has proved invaluable to my clients time and time again is to create a Real Nourishment Menu (to download, go to www.erinharner.com/real-food-resources/). Your Real Nourishment Menu is simply a list of inedible things that you love to do and that nourish your body, mind, and soul. On your nourishment menu, be sure to include things that help you relax or connect like calling a friend, taking a walk, or breathing deeply. This menu is invaluable when you're not hungry and not feeling fulfilled. Many of my clients like to keep their Real Nourishment Menu near the fridge for the weak moments when they are tired, bored, or need something to pick them up. Food won't fill this void, so quit trying—instead of eating, do something that nourishes you from the inside out.

This book is all about creating healthy routines day in and day out because all of your seemingly small choices and actions add up. By forming healthy habits and sticking to them, you create the foundation for health. However ... remember the 90-10 rule? It's okay to break the routine sometimes! Have a glass of wine, enjoy a cup of coffee with a friend, have a piece of dessert. Mixing it up and introducing things that are new and different keeps things interesting and ensures that you don't get stuck in a rut, even a healthy one.

Sometimes, though, we start to slip into old habits. Life happens in cycles. Things come up and you get off track. Don't sweat it, it's normal. The key is to correct your course and get back on track, fast. If you notice that processed foods slowly start to slip back into your diet or you pull through the drive-through for an "emergency" meal because you weren't prepared, chill. It's okay. Just recognize what's going on and remember your *why*. When you eat a diet full of real food, how does it make you feel? Empowered? Healthy? Radiant? Confident?

Getting and staying healthy is a journey. It's a continual process, and you're never done. Start with a few strategies, tips, and tricks in this book. If you try to implement everything that you've learned at once, it can be overwhelming and feel like having a plan is actually making things more complicated. This is a surefire sign that you're moving too fast. Remember, don't try to do everything at once. You can read and revisit this book as often as you want to until you're happy with your progress and your plan. Eating real food and creating a plan for your life before it happens is a long-term solution to being healthy as well as having more energy and less stress. Keep at it and stick with it. It's totally worth it.

If you find that you're having a hard time getting started or making healthy upgrades in your life, get support. Find a coach, nutritionist, doctor, mentor, or friend who can help you figure out what's keeping you stuck, get you moving forward quickly, and provide support to keep you on track to meet your goals. I've given you a lot of strategies in this book to make healthy eating work for you; it's up to you to make it happen.

By having a plan to get you healthy and to keep you healthy, it frees up time and mental energy to focus on what really matters so you can live with renewed inspiration, motivation, and purpose. You've got a plan to be healthy, now go live it up!

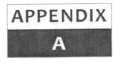

APPENDIX
A

SEASONAL PRODUCE CHART

WINTER (December, January, February)		SPRING (March, April, May)	
VEGETABLES:	**FRUITS:**	**VEGETABLES:**	Mustard greens
Broccoli	Apples	Artichokes	New potatoes
Brussels sprouts	Cranberries*	Asparagus	Peas
Cabbage	Grapefruit*	Avocados*	Spinach
Cauliflower	Kiwis*	Beets	Swiss chard
Collard greens	Lemons*	Broccoli	Watercress
Herbs	Limes*	Carrots	
Kale	Oranges*	Celery	**FRUITS:**
Leeks	Tangerines*	Chives	Cherries
Mushrooms		Collard greens	Mangoes*
Onions		Fennel	Pineapples*
Potatoes		Green onions	Rhubarb
Rutabaga		Herbs	Strawberries
Turnips		Kale	Tangerines*
Winter squash		Lettuces/salad greens	

SUMMER (June, July, August)		FALL (September, October, November)	
VEGETABLES:	Spinach	**VEGETABLES:**	Pumpkins
Beets	Summer squash	Beans	Radishes
Broccoli	Swiss chard	Beets	Spinach
Cabbage	Tomatoes	Broccoli	Sweet potatoes
Carrots	Zucchini	Brussels sprouts	Swiss chard
Celery		Cabbage	Tomatoes
Collard greens	**FRUITS:**	Carrots	Turnips
Corn	Apricots	Cauliflower	Winter squash
Cucumber	Blackberries	Celery	Zucchini
Eggplant	Blueberries	Collard greens	
Garlic	Cherries	Cucumber	**FRUITS:**
Green beans	Melons	Garlic	Apples
Herbs	Nectarines*	Herbs	Cranberries*
Lettuces/salad greens	Peaches	Kale	Figs*
Okra	Pineapples*	Leeks	Grapes
Onions	Plums	Lettuces/salad	Kiwis*
Peas	Raspberries	greens	Melons
Peppers	Strawberries	Mushrooms	Nuts*
Potatoes	Watermelon	Onions	Pears
Radishes		Parsnips	Plums
		Peas	Pomegranates*
		Peppers	Raspberries
		Potatoes	

Produce at its peak but likely not grown locally (unless you live in the Southern U.S.) or imported from outside the United States.

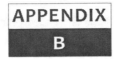

APPENDIX B

SAMPLE REAL-FOOD MEAL PLANS

It's often helpful to see an example when you get started doing something new, and meal planning is no different. If you're struggling with meal planning or just want to get some new ideas, check out these real-food meal plans to get you started making your own. Here are two sample seven-day meal plans— one for summer and one for winter. Each meal plan incorporates a variety of real foods. Simply adapt them to suit your needs and dietary restrictions.

Sample Seven-Day Real-Food Meal Plan for Summer:

Day/#	Breakfast	Lunch	Dinner	Prep Needed
Mon.	Classic oatmeal with berries and walnuts	Black bean, corn, and avocado salad	Grilled salmon with lemon and garlic, vegetable quinoa pilaf	
Tues.	Berry green smoothie	Leftover salmon on salad, vegetable quinoa pilaf	Black bean burgers in lettuce wraps with salsa, sweet potato fries	Soak brown rice for tomorrow's dinner, soak chickpeas
Wed.	Chocolate banana smoothie	Large taco salad with black bean burger, salsa, veggies	Chickpea and lentil dal with brown rice, Swiss chard sauté	Thaw chicken for tomorrow's dinner, freeze extra chickpeas for Sunday
Thurs.	Coconut brown rice pudding using leftover rice	Chickpea and lentil dal with brown rice, Swiss chard sauté	Chicken and veggie fried rice with leftover brown rice	Thaw cod for tomorrow's dinner
Fri.	Fruit and yogurt parfait	Chicken and veggie fried rice, side salad	Baked cod with vegetables, blueberry apple crisp for dessert	Thaw chicken for tomorrow's dinner
Sat.	Blueberry apple crisp with Greek yogurt	Summer picnic quinoa salad	Chicken fajitas with fresh veggies, salsa, black beans	
Sun.	Spinach, onion, and tomato omelet	Summer picnic quinoa salad	Greek salad, falafel with carrot tahini sauce	

Sample Seven-Day Real-Food Meal Plan for Winter:

Day/#	Breakfast	Lunch	Dinner	Prep Needed
Mon.	Leftover toasted buckwheat pancakes with almond butter	Hummus wrap with lettuce, avocado, tomato	Lemon-garlic salmon, green beans amandine, vegetable quinoa pilaf	
Tues.	Coconut-ginger quinoa with almonds and raisins	Leftover lemon-garlic salmon, green beans amandine, vegetable quinoa pilaf	Stove-top veggie chili, cornbread	Soak black beans, make cornbread
Wed.	Classic oatmeal with berries and walnuts	Leftover stovetop veggie chili, cornbread	Black bean and carrot soup, Swiss chard sauté, cornbread	Soak brown rice for tomorrow's dinner
Thurs.	Veggie omelet with Swiss chard, tomatoes, onions, garlic	Leftover black bean and carrot soup, cornbread	Red lentil dal, brown rice, roasted Brussels sprouts	
Fri.	Greek yogurt with Maple nut granola, berries	Leftover red lentil dal, brown rice, roasted Brussels sprouts	Lemon pepper chicken, brown rice risotto, quick 'n' easy kale	
Sat.	Scrambled eggs with leftover quick 'n' easy kale	Lemon-pepper chicken sandwiches	Stuffed peppers with ground turkey and brown rice	
Sun.	Buckwheat pancakes with blueberry sauce	Leftover stuffed peppers with ground turkey and brown rice	Burritos with black beans, lettuce, salsa, avocado, apple crisp	

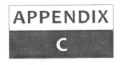

APPENDIX C

REAL–FOOD RECIPES

Here are twenty of my favorite real-food recipes to get you started. Each recipe is simple and delicious. Note that the recipes are organized alphabetically by savory and sweet instead of by category—the Berry Smoothie for example makes a great breakfast, snack, or dessert, and the Quick 'n' Easy Kale makes a great side with dinner or a delicious breakfast omelet filling. These recipes are highly versatile and adaptable, so give them a try and enjoy them!

Savory Real-Food Recipes:

Sweet Real–Food Recipes:

Savory Real–Food Recipes

Balsamic Roasted Beets

Ingredients:
1 bunch beets (about 4 medium), peeled
3 tablespoons balsamic vinegar
3 tablespoons grapeseed oil or olive oil
1/2 teaspoon sea salt

Directions:
Preheat oven to 400 degrees Fahrenheit. Cut beets into 1/4-inch cubes and toss with the vinegar, oil, and sea salt. Pour beets into a 9" x 13" pan and roast for about 40 minutes or until beets are tender.

Black Bean, Corn, and Avocado Salad

Ingredients:
2 cups fresh or frozen corn
1 1/2 cups black beans, cooked
2 cups diced tomatoes
1 onion, finely diced
2 avocados cut into 1/2-inch chunks
1 cup fresh cilantro
1/2 cup flaxseed oil or olive oil
1/2 cup fresh lime juice
2–3 teaspoons finely chopped chili peppers
Sea salt and pepper to taste

Directions:
Cook corn in water for about 2–3 minutes or until crisp-tender. Drain off water and rinse with cold water. Combine corn, beans, tomatoes, onion, avocados, and cilantro in a large bowl. Whisk

oil, lime juice, chili pepper, salt, and pepper in a separate bowl. Pour the dressing over the vegetables and beans, then toss gently to coat. Serve over a bed of lettuce.

Cilantro-Lime Sweet Potato Salad

Ingredients:

4 large sweet potatoes
2 tablespoons oil (olive or grapeseed)
1/3 cup lime juice
2 tablespoons maple syrup (or 8 drops clear stevia)
1/2 cup green onions, chopped
1/4 cup cilantro leaves, chopped
1/2 cup toasted pecans (opt.)
Sea salt and pepper to taste

Directions:

Preheat oven to 400 degrees Fahrenheit. Cut sweet potatoes into 1-inch chunks. Put in a large baking pan, drizzle with 1 tablespoon oil, sprinkle with salt, and mix to coat. Spread potatoes in a single layer and bake, stirring occasionally, until tender when pierced or about 25–30 minutes. In a large bowl, mix lime juice, maple syrup, and remaining oil. Add hot roasted sweet potatoes to lime juice mixture, along with green onions and cilantro. Mix well and season to taste with sea salt and pepper. Top with toasted pecans and serve immediately or store in the fridge until ready to serve.

Crispy Kale Chips

Ingredients:

1 large bunch kale
3 tablespoons olive oil
2 tablespoons toasted sesame oil
2 tablespoons toasted sesame seeds (beige or black)
Sea salt

Directions:

Strip kale off of the stalks and tear it into bite-size pieces. Put the kale and oil in a large bowl and gently massage the oil into the kale. Sprinkle with sesame seeds and sea salt. To make kale chips in a dehydrator, place on dehydrator trays and dehydrate at 115 degrees Fahrenheit for about 2 hours or until kale chips are crispy. To make kale chips in the oven, heat the oven to 400 degrees Fahrenheit, spread kale onto baking sheets, and back for 5 to 8 minutes. Watch very carefully, as kale can burn easily. Remove the kale chips from the oven as soon as they start to turn slightly brown. To keep them fresh, store kale chips in an airtight container, like a glass jar, at room temperature.

Lemon-Garlic Hummus

Ingredients:

1 1/2 cups chickpeas, cooked
1/4 cup sesame tahini
1 tablespoon extra virgin olive oil
2 tablespoons lemon juice
1/2 cup water
2 cloves garlic

1 teaspoon fresh or dried
  parsley
1/4 teaspoon cayenne
  pepper
1/2 teaspoon paprika
pinch sea salt

Directions:

Put all of the ingredients in the food processor or blender and puree until there are no chunks and the mixture is smooth and creamy. Add more water if needed. Transfer to a medium bowl and chill for at least one hour to let the flavors combine before serving. Serve with fresh-cut vegetables.

Lemon-Garlic Grilled Salmon

Ingredients:

2-6oz. wild Alaskan salmon fillets
1 tablespoon grapeseed oil
1 lemon
2 cloves garlic
Sea salt and pepper to taste

Directions:

Light the grill and set to medium-high heat. Put grapeseed oil, juice of half a lemon, and garlic cloves in a blender to combine. Brush salmon on the flesh side with lemon-garlic oil mixture and sear skin side down for about 4 minutes. Brush the flesh side again with the lemon-garlic oil mixture and flip salmon so skin side is up and cook for another 3 to 4 minutes. Remove salmon from the grill and top with remaining lemon-garlic oil mixture. Serve with a wedge of lemon.

Quick 'n' Easy Kale

Ingredients:

1 large bunch kale
2 tablespoons coconut oil (or grapeseed oil)
1 medium onion, chopped
2 cloves garlic, crushed
Sea salt to taste

Directions:

In a medium pot, boil about of 1-inch water. Chop the onion and mince garlic. Wash the kale and strip the leaves from the stems. Compost the stems and cut the leaves into 1/2-inch strips using chiffonade cutting. When the water is boiling, add the kale for about 4 minutes or until the leaves are bright green. In the meantime, sauté the onion in oil until soft, then add garlic and continue sautéing. Add the cooked kale to the onion and garlic sauté and stir to combine. Season to taste with sea salt and serve hot.

Swiss Chard Sauté

Ingredients:

1 large bunch Swiss chard
2 tablespoons grapeseed oil
1 medium onion, chopped
2 cloves garlic, crushed
Sea salt to taste

Directions:

Chop the onion and mince garlic. Wash the Swiss chard and cut the leaves from the stems. Cut the leaves into ½-inch strips using chiffonade. Chop the stems into ½-inch pieces. Sauté the onion in oil until soft, then add garlic and Swiss chard stems and continue sautéing. Add the Swiss chard leaves to the mixture and continue sautéing. Add a bit of water if needed. Season with a pinch of sea salt and serve hot.

Sweet Potato Fries

Ingredients:

3 large sweet potatoes

3 tablespoons grapeseed oil

1–2 tablespoons cane sugar or coconut palm sugar

1 tablespoon sea salt

1–2 tablespoons spice combination of your choice: chipotle powder, paprika, Herbamare, etc.

Directions:

Preheat oven to 450 degrees Fahrenheit. Cut off the ends of sweet potatoes and leave skins on. Cut the sweet potatoes in half lengthwise and then, if they are very long, in half crosswise. Cut each piece into wedges. Put the sweet potatoes into a large bowl and add the oil. Toss to combine. Sprinkle with salt, sugar, and spices of your choice. Use your hands to mix well, so all pieces are coated with oil and spices. Spread the sweet potatoes out in a single layer on a baking sheet; the oil they are coated with should keep them from sticking to the pan. Bake for 25 to 30 minutes. After the first 15 minutes, remove the baking sheet from the oven and turn over all of the sweet potato fries. Return to the oven and bake for another 10–15 minutes or until they are lightly browned and crispy.

Tomato-Cucumber Salad

Ingredients:

2 tomatoes, chopped
1 cucumber, peeled and diced
1 onion, chopped
1 tablespoon lemon juice
1 tablespoon extra-virgin olive oil
Sea salt and pepper to taste

Directions:

Combine tomatoes, cucumbers, and onion in a medium bowl. Toss with oil and lemon juice, then season to taste with salt and black pepper. Chill until ready to serve.

Vegetable Quinoa Pilaf

Ingredients:

2 tablespoons grapeseed oil
1 large onion, chopped
2 stalks celery, chopped
3 carrots, chopped
1 cup quinoa (red or white)

2 cups water or vegetable stock
1 bay leaf
1 tablespoon lemon juice
1 cup frozen peas, thawed
Sea salt and pepper to taste

Directions:

In a medium saucepan, heat oil. Add onion, celery, and carrots and sauté for about 5 minutes or until veggies are crisp-tender. Rinse the quinoa in a fine mesh strainer, drain well, then stir into the vegetables. Add the water or stock, bay leaf, and lemon juice and bring to a boil. Cover, reduce heat to medium-low, and simmer for 15 minutes or until all water is absorbed and quinoa is cooked. Discard the bay leaf, stir in the peas, season with salt and pepper to taste, and serve.

Sweet Real-Food Recipes

Apple Crisp

Ingredients:

3 tablespoons grapeseed oil, divided
4 firm apples, cored and sliced with skins on
2 tablespoons lemon juice
5 tablespoons honey, divided
1 tablespoon cinnamon
2 tablespoons arrowroot starch, corn starch, or flour
1 cup rolled oats
1/4 cup brown-rice flour or other flour
1 tablespoon cinnamon
1/4 cup chopped nuts (walnuts, pecans, or almonds)
Pinch of sea salt

Directions:

Heat the oven to 375 degrees Fahrenheit. Rub 1 tablespoon of oil into an 8" x 8" pan to coat and set aside. Fill the pan with the apples and stir in the lemon juice, 2 tablespoons honey, and cinnamon. You can also use berries, cherries, or peaches mixed in with the apples—get creative. Combine the remaining ingredients in a medium bowl and sprinkle over top of the apples. Bake for 20 to 30 minutes or until the apples are tender and the topping turns golden brown. Serve hot. When cooled, if there is any left, store covered in the fridge.

Berry Green Smoothie

Ingredients:

1/2 cup ice cubes
1/2 cup water
1/2 cup pomegranate juice
1/2 cup frozen berries
1/2 cup fresh spinach, washed
1/4 cup Greek yogurt or protein powder (whey, hemp, brown rice, pea)
1 tablespoon chia seeds or ground flax seeds (optional)

Directions:

Combine all ingredients in a blender and puree until smooth. Add more water if needed to achieve desired consistency. Serve in glasses and enjoy right away.

Chocolate Avocado Pudding

Ingredients:

1 firm avocado
3 teaspoons raw cacao or cocoa powder
2 teaspoons vanilla
2 to 3 tablespoons honey, maple syrup, or 8 drops clear stevia
3 tablespoons water

Directions:

Scoop out avocado and put in blender. Add the remaining ingredients to blender and purée until smooth and creamy. Serve immediately.

Cinnamon-soaked Almonds

Ingredients:

1/2 cup raw almonds
1 cup water
1 teaspoon cinnamon
5 drops clear stevia (optional)

Directions:

In a medium bowl, put the raw almonds in water to soak for 4 to 10 hours and cover with a lid (overnight works best). Drain off the water and add cinnamon and stevia to the almonds. Put in a snack bag or small container to take on the go as a quick healthy snack. Soaked almonds only last a day after soaking them. If you want them to last longer, dehydrate them for 4 to 6 hours at 115 degrees Fahrenheit then store them in an airtight container.

Coconut-Ginger Quinoa

Ingredients:

1 cup quinoa
1 can organic coconut milk
2 tablespoon fresh ginger, grated
2 tablespoons pure maple syrup
1/4 cup raisins (optional)
1/4 cup sliced almonds (optional)
Pinch of salt

Directions:

Rinse quinoa in a fine mesh strainer then boil with 2 cups water. Reduce heat to simmer and cook for 15 minutes. Add coconut milk, ginger, maple syrup, and salt to quinoa and stir. If more liquid is needed, add water, milk, or a milk alternative. Serve for breakfast or dessert and garnish with raisins, almonds, or fresh fruit.

Energy Trail Mix

Ingredients:

1 cup raw walnuts
1 cup raw almonds
1 cup raisins (or dried cranberries)
1 cup raw sunflower seeds
1 cup raw pumpkin seeds
1/2 cup mini chocolate chips or raw cacao nibs (optional)

Directions:

Mix all ingredients together gently. Fill small snack bags with 1/4-cup portions to take with you on the go. You can also add other nuts, seeds, or dried fruit to this trail mix to make it how you'd like or leave out nuts or seeds that you don't like—personalize it.

Fruit and Yogurt Parfait

Ingredients:

1/2 cup fresh fruit (bananas, blueberries, strawberries, apples, grapes, etc.)
1/2 cup plain Greek yogurt
2 tablespoons granola

Directions:

Put some fruit in the bottom of a clear cup or bowl then layer with yogurt, granola, and the rest of the fresh fruit. Serve right away for a great real food breakfast, snack, or dessert.

Maple Nut Granola

Ingredients:

5 cups old-fashioned rolled oats

1 cup raw almonds, chopped

1 cup cashews, chopped

1 cup walnuts, chopped

1 cup sunflower seeds

1 cup pumpkin seeds

1 cup coconut, shredded (optional)

1/2 pure maple syrup

1/2 cup coconut oil

1 cup flax seeds and/or 1/2 cup chia seeds (optional)

1 cup raisins (optional)

Directions:

Preheat the oven to 350 degrees Fahrenheit and line a large baking sheet with parchment paper. Combine all dry ingredients except flax seeds, chia seeds, and raisins in a large bowl. Heat oil and syrup in a small pan over medium heat until melted, then pour over dry ingredients and mix thoroughly. Pour the granola mixture onto the baking sheet, making sure it is a thick layer so that it doesn't burn. Bake for about 20 minutes or until the granola is light brown, and stir a couple times during cooking to prevent burning. Once the granola is cooked, pour into a large bowl, add the raisins, chia seeds, and flax seeds, and allow to cool. Store in an airtight container at room temperature.

Whole-Fruit Sorbet

Ingredients:

2 cups frozen fruit (mangoes, pineapple, peaches, strawberries, bananas, etc.)

1 tablespoon honey (optional)

Directions:

Combine all ingredients in a high-powered blender like a Vitamix or food processor. Blend until smooth and creamy. Top with your favorite toppings like coconut flakes, cacao nibs, raw almonds, or whatever you like, and serve immediately.

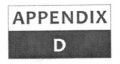

APPENDIX
D

RESOURCES AND SUGGESTED READING

Books on Food and Nutrition:

Animal, Vegetable, Miracle: A Year of Food Life by Barbara Kingsolver

Eat to Live: The Amazing Nutrient-Rich Program for Fast and Sustained Weight Loss, Revised Edition by Joel Fuhrman

In Defense of Food: An Eater's Manifesto by Michael Pollan

The 3-Season Diet: Eat the Way Nature Intended: Lose Weight, Beat Food Cravings, and Get Fit by John Douillard

The China Study: The Most Comprehensive Study Ever Conducted and the Startling Implications for Diet, Weight Loss, and Long-term Health by T. Colin Campbell and Thomas M. Campbell II

The New Optimum Nutrition Bible by Patrick Holford

The Slow Down Diet: Eating for Pleasure, Energy, and Weight Loss by Marc David

Ultrametabolism: The Simple Plan for Automatic Weight Loss by Mark Hyman, MD

What to Eat by Marion Nestle

Real-Food Cookbooks:

Food to Live By: The Earthbound Farm Organic Cookbook by Myra Goodman

How to Cook Everything Vegetarian: Simple Meatless Recipes for Great Food by Mark Bittman and Alan Witschonke

How to Cook Everything: 2,000 Simple Recipes for Great Food by Mark Bittman

The Art of Simple Food: Notes, Lessons, and Recipes from a Delicious Revolution by Alice Waters

The Gluten-Free Almond Flour Cookbook by Elana Amsterdam

The Whole Life Nutrition Cookbook: Whole Foods Recipes for Personal and Planetary Health, Second Edition by Alissa Segersten and Tom Malterre, MS, CN

Online Resources on Food and Nutrition:

Amazon: www.amazon.com
Online retailer with an extensive inventory of hard-to-find food products, gluten-free foods, and organic foods.

Cooperative Grocer Network:
www.cooperativegrocer.coop/coops/
A directory of food cooperatives in the U.S.

Eat Well: www.eatwellguide.org
A directory of locally produced food, farms, stores, and restaurants, searchable by zip code.

Eat Wild: www.eatwild.com/products/
A directory of local grass-fed meat, dairy, and eggs, searchable by state.

Environmental Working Group:
http://www.ewg.org/foodnews/summary/
Non-profit organization that produces the Dirty Dozen Plus™ and Clean 15™ lists based on pesticides in produce.

Got Mercury: www.gotmercury.org
Useful website with a mercury calculator comparing fish consumption to EPA limits and information on mercury contamination in seafood.

Local Harvest: www.localharvest.org
An extensive database of farms, farmer's markets, and CSAs searchable by zip code.

Nutrition Data: www.nutritiondata.com
A database of nutrition information for foods.

Nutrition MD: www.nutritionmd.org
A database of information on how nutrition can play an important role in the prevention and treatment of disease—provided by the Physician's Committee for Responsible Medicine.

Nuts.com: www.nuts.com
Online retailer with a huge inventory of fresh nuts, seeds, dried fruit, and other bulk foods—many of the food items are certified gluten-free and organic.

Seafood Watch: www.seafoodwatch.com
An excellent resource for finding sustainable seafood recommendations.

Acknowledgments

A number of people contributed either directly or indirectly to this book and I'd like to thank you. First, I'd like to thank my parents Chris and Fred, and my siblings Ryan and Chloe. Chloe's design sense and artistic direction was extremely helpful. Also thank you to my extended family for your love and support. And, a special thank you to my amazing husband Dondi for supporting me and believing in me.

Thank you to my coaches Karin Witzig Rozell and Lisa Sarnowski for pushing me and inspiring me to always be my best—because even coaches need coaches! Thank you to my colleagues Mary Langfield-Neaton, Jennifer Boger, and Margitt Royce. Thank you to my professors Diane Dalecki and Amy Lerner for your support and encouragement to pursue my passion.

Thank you to the members of the *Get Real in 8 Weeks Program* for your participation, invaluable input, and feedback to make this a better book: Liz, Chris, Jennifer, Dawn, Cheryl, Peggy, and Jean. And a special thank you to my clients—past, present, and future—for your courage and tenacity to improve your life through real food nutrition. You inspire me every day. This one's for you.

About the Author

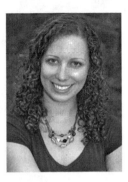 Erin Harner, MS, CHC, is a nutrition coach, popular speaker, nutrition blogger, healthy recipe creator, and your real-food go-to-girl. She received her MS degree in the biomedical sciences from the University of Rochester in Rochester, New York, and studied nutrition at the Institute for Integrative Nutrition in New York City.

Erin is the founder of Healthy Habits International, LLC, a company dedicated to creating optimal health through real food nutrition and functional nutrition. She works with clients individually and in groups, and has a nationwide clientele. Erin lives in Fort Collins, Colorado, with her husband Dondi.

For more information about Erin's products, programs, services, and seminars, go to **www.erinharner.com**.